A History of
Herbalism

A History of Herbalism

Cure, Cook and Conjure

Emma Kay

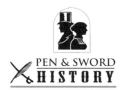

PEN & SWORD
HISTORY

First published in Great Britain in 2022 by
Pen & Sword History
An imprint of
Pen & Sword Books Ltd
Yorkshire – Philadelphia

ISBN 978 1 39900 895 2

A CIP catalogue record for this book is
available from the British Library.

Typeset by Mac Style
Printed and bound in the UK by CPI Group (UK) Ltd,
Croydon, CR0 4YY.

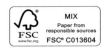

Pen & Sword Books Limited incorporates the imprints of Atlas,
Archaeology, Aviation, Discovery, Family History, Fiction, History,
Maritime, Military, Military Classics, Politics, Select, Transport,
True Crime, Air World, Frontline Publishing, Leo Cooper, Remember
When, Seaforth Publishing, The Praetorian Press, Wharncliffe
Local History, Wharncliffe Transport, Wharncliffe True Crime
and White Owl.

For a complete list of Pen & Sword titles please contact

PEN & SWORD BOOKS LIMITED
47 Church Street, Barnsley, South Yorkshire, S70 2AS, England
E-mail: enquiries@pen-and-sword.co.uk
Website: www.pen-and-sword.co.uk

Or

PEN AND SWORD BOOKS
1950 Lawrence Rd, Havertown, PA 19083, USA
E-mail: Uspen-and-sword@casematepublishers.com
Website: www.penandswordbooks.com

Contents

Acknowledgements

Thanks go out to Alan Murphy at Pen & Sword for having faith in this idea and editor Laura Hirst, as well as all the other staff who work tirelessly putting the proofs together and designing jacket covers and layouts.

Special appreciation to my old and dear friend Rachel Dingsdale for spending a delightful day with me at the Botanical Gardens, Oxford, and sharing in the delights of their wonderful herbarium.

To my gorgeous son and patient husband – thank you both for all your continued support, as ever.

Introduction

The gentian's bluest fringes
Are curling in the sun;
In dusty pods the milkweed
Its hidden silk has spun.[1]

It is quite hard to define a herb; Rosalind Northcote described them thus: 'a herb is a plant, green and aromatic and fit to eat, but it is impossible to deny that there are several undoubted herbs that are not aromatic, a few more grey than green, and one or two unpalatable, if not unwholesome.'[2] So there you have it – the definition, if somewhat vague and incomplete, of a herb in its simplest terms. Many books about

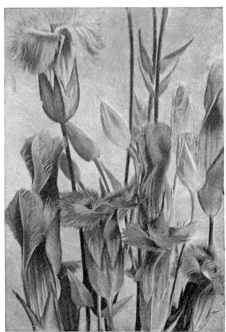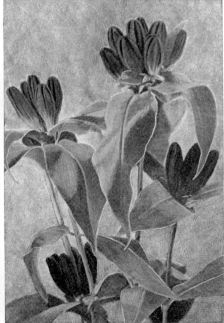

Blue gentians.

herbs tend to include a myriad of miscellaneous plants and all the spices as well. This is probably because spices are often traditionally lumped together with herbs as generic medicines or culinary additions. Whilst you may find reference to some plants and roots which are not strictly herbs in this book, you will not find any information relating to spices. I wanted this to be a book that focused specifically on the properties of herbs where possible.

The World Health Organization (WHO) refers to herbs as 'herbal materials, herbal preparations, and finished herbal products that contain whole plants, parts of plants, or other plant materials, including leaves, bark, berries, flowers, and roots, and/or their extracts as active ingredients intended for human therapeutic use or for other benefits in humans and sometimes animals'.[3]

I find classifying is essential to understanding herbs and throughout this book you will discover the wide and complex use of plants in magic, cooking and medicine, the three areas that made the most sense to me in terms of herbology.

In 1895 a remarkable thing happened. Alicia Amherst published a list of herbs that she cited as belonging to the fifteenth century, from a manuscript unearthed within the pages of an old cookery book. Since then, several researchers have identified this comprehensive list as likely to have been compiled around the beginning of the 1500s, with the handwriting consistent of that used within the reign of Henry VIII. They also identified a potential author, as one Thomas Fourmond, or Fromond, who was the owner of land in both Carshalton and Cheam. He died around 1542.[4] The 'Fromond list' was reclassified by John Harvey in 1989, according to Alicia's original list, which was then comprehensively reformatted by the historic gardener and author Sylvia Landsberg in 2003.

To me this list provides a useful guide to English medieval herb classification, representing a timeless approach to indexing the various properties of herbs, their uses and character.

Herbs for pottage
Agrimony, Alexanders, astrologia longa, A. rotunda, avens, basil, beet, betony, borage, cabbage, caraway, chervil, chives, clary, colewort, columbine, coriander, daisy, dandelion, dill, dittander, fennel, good king henry, hart's-tongue, langdebeef, leek, lettuce, lupin, mallow, marigold

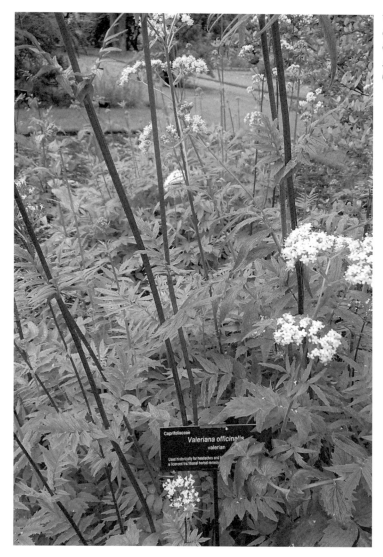

Valerian at
Oxford Botanic
Garden and
Arboretum.
(*Emma Kay*)

(pot), marjoram, mint, nepp, nettle (red), oculus Christi, orach, parsley, patience, pepperwort, radish, rape, safflower, sage, spinach, thistle, milk, thyme, valerian, violet, wood sorrel, (sowthistle).

Herbs for sauce
Dittander, harts-tongue, masterwort, mints, parsley, pellitory, sorrel, violet, (garlic mustard), (wood sorrel).

Herbs for the cup (for infusing in water or wine)
Carnation, clary, cost, costmary, endive, hyssop, marjoram, marigold (pot), rosemary, rue, chamomile, horehound.

Herbs for salad
Alexanders, borage, calamint, chickweed, chives, cress (French), daisies, dandelion, fennel, heartsease, mints, nettle (red), parsley, primrose buds, purslane, rampion, ramsons, rocket, violets, burnet, cresses.

Herbs to distil
Betony, dragons (tarragon), endive, eyebright, hyssop, mugwort, rose (red), rosemary, sage, scabious, silverweed, water pepper, wormwood.

Roots and bulbs
Carrots, eryngo, parsnips, radish, saffron, turnips, (onions).

Herbs to taste and/or smell
Basil, carnation, dropwort, dill, garlic, germander, marjoram (sweet), melons, poppy (garden), Solomon's seal, vervain, (wallflower).

Herbs for a herber or ornamental garden
Trees: almond, bay, peach, pine, plum; Shrubs: gooseberry, gourds, roses (white), vine; Herbaceous plants: campion, columbine, cornflour, hellebore, lilies, peony (roman), safflower.[5]

As Fromond's list suggests, with names like 'Good King Henry', hart's-tongue, masterwort and silverweed, so many herbs and plants, once revered and praised for their therapeutic and curative abilities, have been lost from our diets. Goosefoot, which does not appear on the Fromond list but was also known as fat hen, pigweed and lambs' quarters, can be eaten raw in salads or cooked like spinach and has been consumed since Neolithic times. Whilst still popular across Asia and southern Africa, it somehow lost its charm in northern Europe, although its favoured family member, quinoa, is now eaten widely everywhere.

Goosefoot, so called because its leaves are shaped like that of a goose, belongs to the amaranth family, and writing in 1597, John Gerard informs us that it grew abundantly, but was never considered to have any medicinal value. Rather, its leaves, were regularly added to salads. Gerard also points out that it was known to be poisonous to pigs.[6]

Quinoa is a species of goosefoot. Similar to buckwheat, quinoa was valued for its nutritional attributes during the Victorian period. Once the staple diet of Peruvians, the seeds were initially considered a little unpalatable to European and American tastes, who preferred to boil the young shoots and stems, serving them as an alternative to asparagus. The young quinoa leaves were also added to salads, while older leaves were devoured as boiled greens.[7]

You would also be hard pushed to find a medieval English recipe book that omits the flowering tansy. Fashioned into cakes or fried egg dishes, this herb was also thought to be extremely useful in alleviating a host of medical issues as well as repelling insects. Today, most people would not even recognize the name.

In earlier times borage was cultivated in abundance and employed as a healer of wounds. You can find numerous culinary recipes of the past in which this ginseng-like herb features. (See Chapter 3 to get some ideas of how to utilize borage.) Chickweed – of which there are many varieties – was a plant known for its ability to ease eczema, or in a more ancient capacity, as a motivator of birds to hatch. Sorrel was integral to the preparation of salads, sauces and vinegars, while mugwort, along with agnus castus, could counteract tiredness. Another disregarded herb, rue, is strong scented and was widely believed to protect people from snake and spider bites, bees, hornets and wasps. Long-discarded figwort could keep you healthy if worn around the neck, while versatile angelica acted as a shield against witchcraft.[8]

The snapdragon – so called for when pressed open, it resembles the mouth of a creature which is biting or snapping – was also once highly valued for resisting witchcraft and its leaves were sometimes used to relieve tumours and ulcers. In Russia, the snapdragon was at one time abundantly cultivated for its oil which was by all accounts comparable to olive oil.[9] These florae represent just a small sample of preloved and multifunctional plants that have become redundant.

Early Greek physicians recorded extensive lists of herbs and their restorative powers before the Romans came along with their strange magical and pagan notions of medicine. It was Greek physician Galen of Pergamon, with his legitimization of Hippocrates' 'four humors' that established the first recognized science of anatomy, culminating in an extended period where all other related ancient texts were abandoned.

Hippocrates, or 'the father of medicine', took Plato's notions of the four classical elements: earth, air, water and fire and created the 'four humors'. Hippocrates' four humeral theories are as follows: blood (the air element) being hot and moist; phlegm (the water element) which is cold and moist; yellow bile (the fire element) which is hot and dry; and black bile, or the earth element, which is cold and dry. The theory behind this is the need for both the humors and elements to remain balanced throughout the body in order to maintain general wellness. Additional plants and herbs were

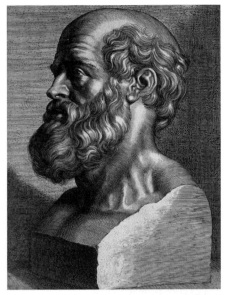

Hippocrates.

applied accordingly to restore any imbalances. For example, if your blood pressure was high, or you had too much yellow bile, a cooling herb such as sage might be administered.

The most universally recognized form of herbal medicine is that which originated in China. Chinese herbal science was born out of a broad philosophy of both masculine yang and feminine yin, the latter hot and powerful, the former cold and yielding, each combining with the five elements relating to water, fire, earth, metal and wood – a similar take on Hippocrates' black bile, yellow bile, phlegm and blood. Red plants were fiery and used to combat fevers; think of the old idiom of fighting fire with fire. Liquids extracted from yellow plants were considered compatible with kidney conditions, while anything heart-shaped, including the leaves or bulbs, were rationalized as being healthy to the heart and pulse.[10]

Shen nong Ben cao jing (*The Divine Farmers' Materia Medica*) is a compilation of three volumes of oral histories recorded in third-century China. It is understood to be the first traceable authority on medicine which categorized well over 300 herbs into three separate groups: upper (harmless to humans), middle (therapeutic but potentially toxic) and lower (those that are poisonous). For example, *Angelica biserrata*, from the Angelica family, was considered non-toxic and was used to relieve pain as well as something dubbed 'running piglet', a term referring to heart palpitations and anxiety – akin to a small pig running around inside your body.[11]

While China developed their herbal remedies, other cultures like the Sumerians (modern-day Iraq) were recording their recipes on clay tablets.[12]

There are tablets belonging to Yale University's Babylonian Collection with detailed inscriptions for culinary recipes, deemed the oldest-known recipes in the world. Three of these tablets come with a date of circa 1730 BC, the fourth being around 1,000 years later. All originate from the Mesopotamian region. One lists the ingredients for twenty-five different stews and broths. Jean Bottéro was a French historian who specialized in Mesopotamian archaeology, researching, writing and lecturing about

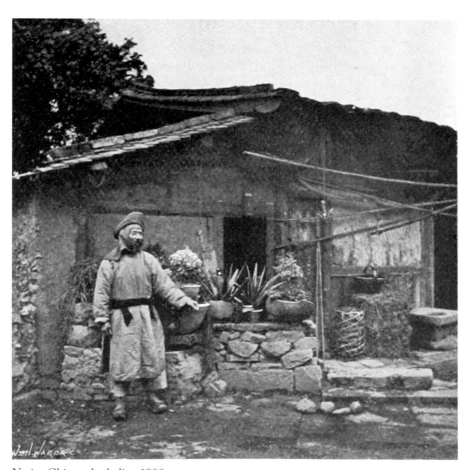

Native Chinese herbalist, 1800s.

these ancient culinary tomes. In his 1987 paper, 'The Culinary Tablets at Yale', Bottéro noted that the most popular supplementary ingredients for almost all the recipes included leeks, onions and garlic. In addition, cumin, coriander and juniper berries featured regularly, as did mint. The tablets contain intricate cooking instructions including the following translated vocabulary: mixing, slicing, squeezing, shredding, crumbing, straining and filtering. Bottéro's research paper also contains several translated complete recipes, like this for raised turnips:

> Meat is not needed. You set water. You throw fat in … Onion, dorsal thorn (unknown), coriander, cumin and kanasu (unknown), leek and garlic, which you squeeze together and spread on the dish. Onion and mint which you add to the crock.[13]

It is difficult to comprehend that these elaborate recipes and instructions belong to communities living 4,000 years ago and to appreciate how keenly they relied on basic vegetables and herbs.

The Sumerians brewed special liquors made from herbs and grains. These beers are recorded in the *Epic of Gilgamesh* and were drunk throughout the day on a daily basis. *Gilgamesh* is an epic Mesopotamian text, compiled in the second millennium BC, with the eponymous hero's challenges and adventures charted across several narratives. In the story of 'The Magic Plant', Gilgamesh seeks out the plant, which some modern translators have likened to buckthorn, in order to restore and rejuvenate his life force. Lured by the surroundings of paradise, Gilgamesh takes his eyes off the plant for a moment, providing an opportunistic snake with a nice green dinner. The symbolic snake then sheds its skin. It has received the benefits of rejuvenation and not mankind. There are numerous tales in European folk literature alluding to the ancient Greek legend of one serpent spying on its friend being killed, before leaving the site and then returning with a special herb that it presses against its dead friend, immediately restoring the snake back to life.[14] All these stories emphasize the extent to which plants were venerated, as nature's way of restoring one's health and well-being.

The *Libellus de Medicinalibus Indorum Herbis* (*Little Book of the Medicinal Herbs of the Indians*) or, more commonly known as the *Badianus Manuscript* is an Aztec herbal, originally translated in 1552, but which fell into the hands of many others and has been translated several times since. The Mexican plant life within this manuscript was categorized as either woody or herbaceous. These were then sub-categorized as edible, medicinal, ornamental or economic. The text of the *Badianus Manuscript* is beautifully illustrated, and is composed of sixty-three folios divided into thirteen chapters which group together a variety of ailments and remedies. The following remedy for catarrah, called Gravedo from the translation of Emily Wollcott, follows:

> **Gravedo**
> *Qui narium distillation seu coriza infestatur herbas atochietl, et Tzompili-huizxihuitl olfaciet et ita gravedini subveniet* (those troubled with a dripping nose or cold are to sniff the herbs Atochietl and tzompilihuizxihuitl and help the cold thus).[15]

Crossing the ancient continents again, Japanese traditional medicine is known as Kampo and it works on the premise that the mind and gut are inseparable. It is also based on many of the same principles as Chinese medicine and is woven into the fabric of the Japanese contemporary health care system. Shiso is a Japanese herb from the mint family with all the flavours of citrus, basil and coriander, to name a few. Typically, shiso is used widely in Japanese cooking, particularly in sushi, tempuras and sashimi dishes. Japanese parsley, or mitsuba, has the taste and look of parsley, but it is also similar to celery and is primarily used as a garnish or an addition to soups. The first edition of the *Japanese Pharmacopoeia* was published in the 1800s and in 2016 an English version was made available. Essentially it is an official document listing all the criteria for and necessary testing of medicines in Japan and includes complex WHO guidelines for assessing the quality of herbal medicines. Many plants are listed in the *Pharmacopoeia* inclusive of Ephedra, which has been known to be fatal, the geranium herb or herb-Robert, known to treat diarrhoea and issues with the liver amongst others. There are also herbs including Leonurus or mother-wort, which has European folklorist connections with protection from evil spirits, mint and plantain.[16]

In 2002, the World Health Organization reported that around 80 per cent of people in Africa relied on traditional medicine. Many parts of rural Africa continue to rely on traditional healers who prescribe medicinal plants that are both affordable and readily accessible. For many African communities, traditional healers also provide counselling, family guidance and an individual level of treatment developed out of a personal understanding of the patient's environment and circumstances. Herbal remedies including wormwood, of which the leaves or bark are considered valuable to sufferers of diabetes, rooibos for cholic, honeybush for chronic catarrh, Umckalaobo (African geranium) for acute respiratory infections and so on.[17]

Herbs have been used medicinally for thousands, if not millions of years. Some of the first recorded are those used by the Egyptians. Herbs were placed in lodestones, which are magnetic mineral rocks and these rocks were then applied to various parts of the body, along with spices, herbal drinks and the burning of herbs to assist with curing diseases and healing a variety of illnesses.[18]

Interestingly, the Egyptians, as ratified in one of the oldest medical herbals of ancient Egypt, the *Ebers Papyrus*, maintain the theory that 'every disease to which men are liable, is occasioned by the substances whereon they feed', meaning there was once little distinction between edible food plants and medicinal plants. Dating to around 1500 BC, but authenticated as much earlier, this medical herbal is named after the Egyptologist Georg Ebers and contains around 700 remedies and formulas.

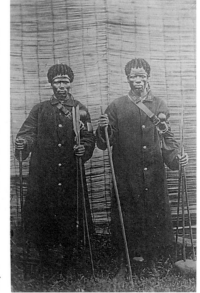

Diseases in ancient Egypt were interpreted as demons that required an exorcism and medicine was just one branch of magic with which to exorcize them. Incantations to expel evil spirits were varied and complex and were categorized as the Maklu (burning), Ti'i (headaches), Asakki marsuti (fever), Labartu (hag-demon) and Nis kati (raising of the hand) One of these incantation reads:

Arise ye great gods, hear my complaint, Grant me justice, take cognizance of my condition.

African witchdoctors, 1882.

I have made an image of my sorcerer and sorceress.
I have humbled myself before you and bring to you my cause,
Because of the evil they have done,
Of the impure things which they have handled.
May she die! Let me live!
May her charm, her witchcraft, her sorcery be broken.
May the plucked sprig of the binu tree purify me.
May it release me; may the evil odor of my mouth be scattered to
    the winds.
May the Mashtakal herb [probably soapwort] which fils the earth
    cleanse me.
Before you let me shine like the kankal herb,
Let me be brilliant and pure as the lardu herb.

Similar perhaps to Africa, India also had its physician-sages. The *Ayurveda* (*Knowledge of Life*) is a book of collected Hindu teachings containing the botanical and spiritual principles of Indian medicine. The ancient Indian text *RigVeda* tells us that herbs were present some three eras before the Gods were even born. It cites over 1,000 medicinal plants.

The *Ayurveda*, like that confirmed by so many other cultures, highlights the importance of the five elements: earth, air, fire, water and ether (the element that was once thought to occupy the upper regions of space). It was essential for these energies to maintain their balance or a person's health became compromised. Cool, calming herbs such as chamomile were used to soothe the stomach; cinnamon and nutmeg could increase a person's stamina, while ginger, cardamom and turmeric were considered ideal for stabilizing the body as a whole.[19]

The Romans made great efforts to acclimatize and cultivate new plants and herbs in England. The earliest books on herbs and their properties relied on translating the works of famous Greek and Roman botanists like Dioscorides and Pliny, together with the studies of Arabic physicians. But these were simply inspired by even earlier ancient theories, particularly those that recorded the healing of animals – birds and other beasts, creatures who ingested herbs to counteract poisons. Archaic texts inform us that scorpions ate white hellebore as an antidote to aconite, weasels ate rue before engaging in combat, hawks applied the juice of hawkweed and swallows celandine to restore the eyesight of their young.[20]

Very early healers believed spirits lived in plants, rocks and flowers and, by actively investigating some of these things, they learnt that certain roots, herbs, berries and leaves were able to stave off pain and some illnesses. In the Middle Ages, the planets, particularly Saturn, Jupiter, Mars, Venus, Mercury and the sun and moon, were celestial bodies thought to possess their own personalities. Pick up any western European book on herbs right up until the nineteenth century and you will find that many, if not most, correlated the properties of herbs directly to specific planets. In medieval art some planets were depicted with human features or personified in human form.[21]

As such, the planets were integral to astrology and the pseudoscience of astrological signs. *Pseudo-Apuleius* is the name given to *Pseudo-Apuleius Herbarius* or *Herbarium Apuleii Platonici*, which attributes this fourth-century text to the Roman poet, Apuleius of Madaura. Many scholars have refuted its provenance believing it instead to be the work of several different authors. In his *Philosophy of Natural Magic*, sixteenth-century German occultist and scholar Cornelius Agrippa von Nettesheim discusses the way in which herbs are aligned to specific signs and plants within the text of *Apuleius*.

These include sage to Aries, straight-growing vervain to Taurus, bending vervain to Gemini, comfrey to Cancer, sow-bread (cyclamen) to Leo, calamint to Virgo, mugwort to Libra, scorpion-grass (forget-me-nots) to Scorpio, pimpernel to Sagittarius, docks to Capricorn, dragon's-wort (tarragon) to Aquarius and hartwort (a Mediterranean herb) to Pisces.[22]

The planets and how they aligned influenced the four elements within the body. Zodiac charts were used to make a diagnosis and whichever astrological sign you were born under also played a part in what treatment you received. There was superstition with herbs; some needed to be gathered at special hours of the day and at different lunar cycles, and even the way they were plucked, be it up or down, could affect their healing powers.

Magic in early medieval Europe specifically involved the process of either harming or controlling. The oldest surviving English herbal is Bald's *Leechbook*, which dates to the tenth century.

As well as the monasteries, both travelling and native herbalists served the communities, with folk medicine being a common practice within every home. The most popular herbs used to guard against witchcraft, often found to be hanging in people's doorways and houses in Elizabethan times, were vervain, dill and rowan.[23] There were all manner of strange pagan and demonic beliefs, many of which are included in the *Leechbook*. 'Elf sickness' was something that took over a person quickly, leaving them weak and incapacitated. There were numerous charms to counteract it. Invisible wounds could be created by supernatural forces; e.g. an injury, such as an arrow which was shot by an elf, could make a person or indeed an animal sick. According to Bald's *Leechbook*, if a horse was injured in this way, the necessary remedy involved a mixture of sorrel seeds and something called 'Scottish wax', mixed with holy water, accompanied by the singing of twelve masses.[24]

Throughout the 'Dark Ages' monasteries were at the centre of all intellectual and academic activity and as such they acted as early infirmaries with medicinal plant gardens on site to treat patients. These treatments were largely based on information passed down from Greek or Roman physicians, like Dioscorides.

There are numerous historical professions linked to the legacy of herbology in England. The Barber Surgeons' Company, a merging of barbers and surgeons, has its roots in the 1300s, while the Society of Apothecaries was established as late as 1617, but evolved out of the much earlier Pepperers' Guild and Grocers' Company of the medieval period.

Apothecaries, who were a mighty force within the Company of Grocers, hocked a range of medicines from herbal remedies to chemical treatments. The College of Physicians, the earliest official English medical society, regulated the barber-surgeons and the apothecaries. The prosecutions of both were infinite throughout the Elizabethan era. The medieval English philosopher Thomas Hobbes declared that he would 'rather have the advice or take physic from an experienced old woman that had been at many sick people's bedsides, than from the learnedest but unexperienced physician'.[25]

The earliest medicinal practitioners were indeed the herbalists, yarbs, wortcunners, witchdoctors, wise women and sorcerers. Today we would label them as homeopathic or alternative. Yarb is a word for herbs or a herbalist particularly associated with the Midlands and the North of

England, as well as the West Country. These herb gatherers were also sometimes called 'simples'.

There was a time when most people possessed a general knowledge of medicinal herbs, when doctors were scarce and pharmacies were non-existent. Acquiring a knowledge of herbal properties and their healing powers gradually became less and less important with the onset of modern medicine. In former times anyone could practise medicine without a licence or a diploma. Herbology, blood-letting, poulticing and blistering were the primary treatments for all manner of ills.

You will find in this book a section dedicated to numerous men and women who played a significant role within the overall historic narrative of British herbs and herbology. Two other notable figures that I would like to mention here include Jean Baptista van Helmont, who was the first person to teach the chemistry of the human body. Christened the 'Descartes of Medicine', he recognized the process of human digestion before anyone else. Born in 1577, he dedicated his life to alchemy and claimed to have seen and touched the infamous 'philosopher's stone'. Several hundred years before Helmont, Pietro d'Abano from Padua, a thirteenth-century philosopher, astrologer and man of medicine practised occult-related sciences. D'Abano lived and studied in Turkey and Paris before being tried for heresy back in his native Padua. He died before a second inquiry found him guilty, but friends recovered his body ahead of the authorities violating his remains according to his sentence. Among his written works scholars tend to attribute d'Abano to the book of *Heptameron*, or magical elements. He believed that magical rites were best performed alongside the burning of fragrant herbs and aromatic spices.[26]

These are just two examples, illustrating the blurred lines between mythology and medicine, folklore and science. Throughout history all these elements are intwined within the wider chronology of the theoretical and practical administration of herbs.

Before the male-dominated guilds monopolized the long-standing successful relationship that women had with midwifery, one of the first significant European texts on women's medicine appeared in the twelfth century in Salerno in Italy which was at the time widely understood to be the most important centre of medicine in Europe, largely due to its acceptance of Arabic philosophies. The text is often attributed to the female healer, Trota of Salerno. Trota advocated the use of opiates and herbs in childbirth to relieve pain and encourage a smoother delivery. Sadly, the abilities of early female midwives like Trota generated suspicion and the Church soon began to place a stop on unregulated female physicians who had the power to assist during labour, administering charms and unlicensed skills.

In what has generically become known simply as *Trotula*, this ensembled work, the origins of which can be traced to an Arabic manuscript and the musings of Muslim women based in Sicily, together with Trota's theories, the text refers to pains in the womb as a consequence of a miscarriage or 'menstrual retention' akin to excessive 'cold' or 'heat'. If cold, the symptoms were likely to manifest as sharp stabbing pains. If hot, the genital area would burn, which was often blamed on extreme sexual activity. Hot herbs were used to treat cold symptoms and cold herbs for hot symptoms, with the exception of marshmallow, traditionally known as a 'cold' herb which was applied to women considered 'frigid'.[27]

In England during the first quarter of the fifteenth century, King Henry V ordered a ban on all female practitioners of medicine, with

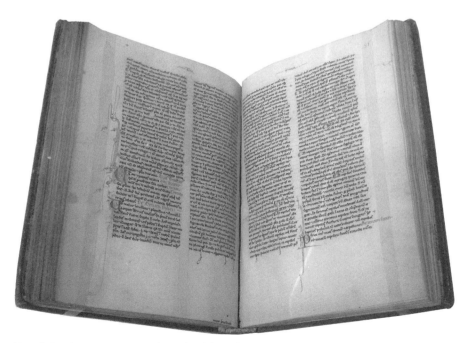

Trotula De Ornatu Mulierum from the fifteenth century.

the English Parliament legislating 'no woman was to use the practice of fysyk'.[28]

Greater suspicion befell women on the instructions of men and men's own fears of female empowerment. In the latter part of the Middle Ages female healers were persecuted for witchcraft. Rumours circulated of their collaboration with Satan himself, and possessing the powers of sorcery, which they applied to their healing practices. Some early manuals on midwifery accused midwives of witchcraft. Hiltprand's textbook of midwifery in the 1500s, branded those women who assisted during births which resulted in stillborn or disabled infants, as witches.[29]

The *Malleus Maleficarum* or the *Hammer of Witches* was written by the clergy and published in Germany in the 1400s. At the time it strongly influenced the culture of torturing and killing witches throughout Europe. It stipulated that 'No one does more harm to the Catholic Faith than midwives. For when they do not kill children, then, as if for some other purpose, they take them out of the room and, raising them up in the air, offer them to devils', stating that 'devils employ certain lower bodies, such as herbs, stones, animals, and certain sounds and voices, and figures'.[30]

Between the fifteenth and seventeenth centuries in western societies, knowledge of herbal medicine was hugely widespread, largely due to the amount of printed material that was being circulated, although it must also be remembered that it was only accessible to the literate. The first two popularist herbals were compiled by John Gerard and Nicholas Culpeper, although the former was largely plagiarized. Conviction in the use of herbs medicinally was queried during the seventeenth century when they proved ineffective during the Great Plague of London. By the next century with the Dawn of Enlightenment, people's attitudes towards superstitions, omens, fairies and all other magical practices began to decline, largely as a consequence of science, freethinking and changes in attitude. However, in places like the new colonies of the Americas herbals were still heavily relied upon for their medical knowledge, with trained physicians being scarce.

The biomedical science of pharmacology emerged in the nineteenth century, which basically forged a formal understanding of how drugs directly impacted on the body. However, herbalists like the American

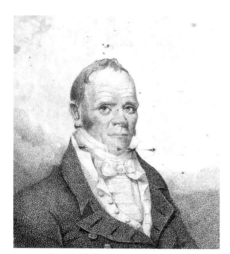

Samuel Thomson, creator of the Thomsonian system.

Samuel Thomson continued to revive accepted herbal practices across both sides of the Atlantic.

And movements like the 'Eclectic physicians' offered herbal treatments as an alternative to some of the nineteenth century's persistent primitive methods of leeches and mercury, two prevalent methods for example, of treating sexually transmitted diseases. Another medicinal concept that was common throughout many countries in Europe, right up to the 1800s, was the notion that diseases could be transmitted from a human to an animal. Hence feeding a dog bread that contained the sweat of a sick man or woman could remove the illness, a treatment which has its roots in medieval nostrums.

New legislation enforced in the twentieth century prevented herb doctors from performing, including the regulation of all medicines, which was updated in the early part of the noughties. However, 'traditional' herbal medicines, which comply with quality standards considered beneficial to conditions like coughs and colds or rheumatic pains, remain on the market.

As of 2018, a total of thirty-four member states across the six WHO regions included 'traditional or herbal medicines in their national essential medicines lists'. Other member states, such as Ghana, had their own separate list of essential herbal medicines. However, over 50 per cent of the WHO member states had also developed the improved regulation of herbal remedies and recognized the importance of the role of integrating new health systems in the same year.[31]

Today the market for alternative medicine continues to boom. In 2016, the global herbal medicine market was valued at a staggering US$71.9 billion and is expected to continue growing.[32] In a world where the delivery of modern medicine is either limited or stretched beyond its capacity, it is perhaps unsurprising that so many people continue to refer to more natural forms of treatment and self-diagnosis. It is after all inherent in the very fabric of our primal beings.

Whilst I do not advocate the sole use of herbal and other alternative methods of healing for serious or life-threatening conditions, I certainly tend to consult natural options for minor ailments and illnesses as a starting point and have discovered that there is a tremendous correlation between the gut and the brain. Lavender, sage, the root of black cohosh and chamomile are staple remedies in our house, as is the mineral selenium, plus I grow countless culinary herbs to access daily. In a society that has become so dependent on processed food, we all, as a family, regularly indulge in a cocktail of high-strength natural yeasts in the form of probiotics to repair the gut, a modern equivalent to the fermented foods we all once consumed in abundance.

Magic and witchcraft may no longer actively play a role in society, but the way I see it, there is more than ever before, a desire to reclaim what has been lost from our environments and a shift towards understanding better the properties of nature to enhance our health, well-being and spiritual happiness. Writing this book has not only encouraged me to grow more herbs, but it has also inspired me to experiment and engage with new herbs in cooking as well as for mild medicinal purposes.

Herbs have beguiled, charmed, restored, benefitted, confused, terrified and influenced societies in countless ways for thousands of years; they should be venerated, cultivated wherever possible and never taken for granted.

With the exception of Nicholas Culpeper, who died of tuberculosis and a couple of other unlucky individuals, all the key herbalists cited in this book lived extraordinarily long lives for the times in which they lived, testament perhaps to the medicinal virtues that they pedalled.

Chapter 1

From 'Witches' to Botanists: British Pioneers, Popularists and Everyday Herbalists

I do remember an apothecary –
And hereabouts a dwells – which late I noted
In tattered weeds, with overwhelming brows,
Culling of simples. Meagre were his looks.
Sharp misery had worn him to the bones,
And in his needy shop a tortoise hung,
And alligator stuffed, and other skins
Of ill-shaped fishes; and about his shelves
A beggarly account of empty boxes,
Green earthen pots, bladders, and musty seeds,
Remnants of packthread, and old cakes of roses
Were thinly scattered to make up a show.[1]

Before the birth of modern medicine, every culture, religion and community relied on either their own knowledge, or the expertise of a practitioner who knew how to treat a spectrum of ailments. This involved gathering herbs, spices, and plants, reciting incantations, rituals and charms, and mixing various organic and inorganic substances, based on a prior and inherent understanding of learned practises passed down from generation to generation. The oldest surviving English herbal medical text is *Bald's Leechbook*, Bald himself being a doctor or 'leech', whose work was founded in Anglo-Saxon traditions and folklore. A salve for the treatment of eye infections made from onions, garlic and samples of a cow's stomach, which Bald included in his manuscript, was legitimized several years ago when scientists from the University of Nottingham were astonished to find that it almost completely eradicated the bacteria MRSA during a series of experiments.[2]

What this conveys is perhaps a need to understand better the principles of ancient medicine, opposed to disregarding it as mythical quackery.

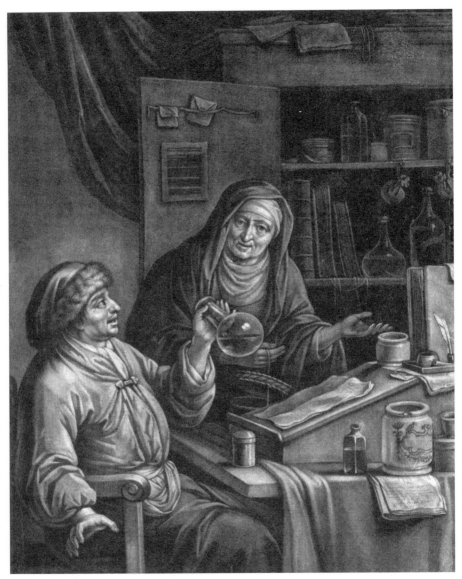

Print made by Bernard Lens, 1659–1725, British, after Adriaen Verdoel, c.1620–c. 1692, Dutch, *An Apothecary*, undated, Mezzotint on moderately thick, moderately textured, cream laid paper. (Yale Center for British Art, Paul Mellon Fund, B1970.3.1046)

Somewhere that natural medicines remain utilized and respected widely, is in Africa. Traditional healers have been working within their own communities for thousands of years. They are recognized, established and trusted figures. In fact, in many areas around the world where orthodox medicine is inaccessible or distrusted, traditional medicine prevails.

As with Africa and elsewhere, every village in Britain once had a herbalist, referred to in some parts of the country as a 'yarb', to minister basic herbal treatments for the sick and injured. Some gathered herbs which they prepared as ointments, tinctures, even snuff. Others cultivated medicinal plants in their own gardens to treat neighbours and the community and there were writers who catalogued and offered early literal society a wealth of knowledge relating to the pharmaceutical benefits of plants, based on the legacy of ancient scholars.

Unlike spices, most herbs were cultivated in the UK, some of which we can thank the Romans for, some the French, some, Scandinavia. Coriander seeds: yes, technically a herb and not a spice, would have been one of the few exceptions, imported as early as the 1500s via Antwerp.

So, who were the characters who researched, wrote about and dispensed these therapeutic potions and lotions? What are their stories? How did they learn their craft and what reputations did they secure? When it came to medicine and understanding the necessities of the human mind and body, most evolving Western cultures relied on earlier written authorities. These came in the form of the great Greek and Roman scholars and philosophers. Hippocrates and his collated medical treatises documented in *Corpus*, Galen and his four temperaments: Sanguine, Choleric, Melancholic and Phlegmatic, the musings of Diocles Medicus or Pliny's *Natural History*. The Greek physician and botanist Pedanius Dioscordes wrote a pharmacopeia called *De Materia Medica* circa AD 50, which was translated into English in 1655 by John Goodyer. It was considered to be one of the greatest authorities on medicine. It was not particularly original – merely a compendium of herbs and plants that were already known throughout the Roman Empire – but it laid the foundations of botany and the direct link between it and medicine. Scholars throughout the Renaissance and beyond continued to refer to Dioscorides.

But communities also looked to the East for medicinal inspiration. Muslim physician Ibn Khatimah recommended cultivating well-stocked gardens with cool plants, like myrtle, to protect your household from pestilence. Having been witness to a plague that swept through Andalusia in the 1340s, he equated foul and infected air with the contagion. Ibn's thinking was founded in much earlier Islamic beliefs in purifying the air

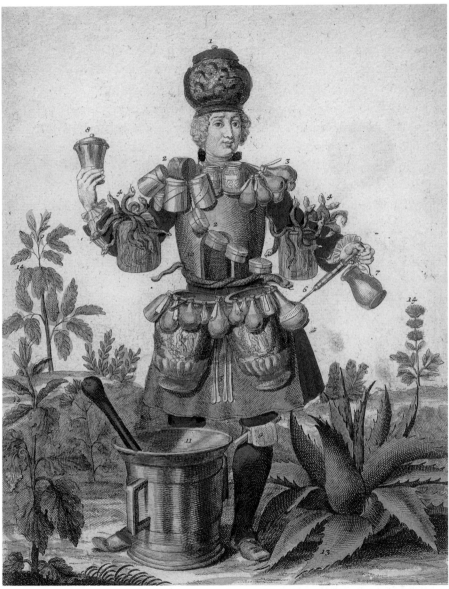

An apothecary with the tools, costume and apparatus. This file comes from Science Museum Group, in the United Kingdom (archive). (*Wellcome Collection L0028713*)

with sweet-smelling plants, strewing herbs indoors and generally across the floors of overcrowded areas.[3] One of the predominant scholars of the Arabian school of medicinal botany was Avicenna (Ibn Sina), who wrote the five-book compilation, *The Canon of Medicine*. It was completed in the early part of the eleventh century and was used as a standard textbook for medicine across both Medieval Europe and the Islamic world. It explored physiology and the nature of contagious diseases, investigating the notion of quarantine.

Revered early medieval physician Constantine the African, who is thought to have died sometime in the late tenth century, was probably an Arab Muslim who emigrated to Italy where he wrote lengthy medicinal texts based on his own extraordinary knowledge of Arabic medicine. As such he was one of the first to be credited with broadening the evolving European panacea. Constantine is most associated with the study of aphrodisiacs and claimed (or rather, boasted) to have tried and tested them all.[4]

Allegedly J. Falcand de Luca was the first officially recorded apothecary granted permission to sell medicines in England, in 1357.

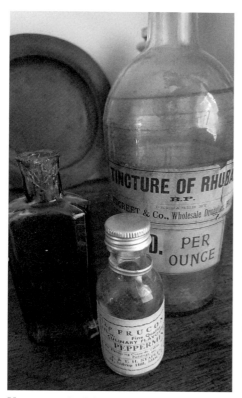

There were clearly earlier traders as the archives mention shops like that of Master Otto of Germany, 'a physician of repute', who sold medicinal compounds from his shop in York in 1292.

Apothecaries evolved from the Guild of Pepperers, a company of merchant traders who imported a range of medicinal wares and culinary spices, first mentioned around the twelfth century. By the fourteenth century the rather long-winded fraternity known as the Pepperers or Easterlings of Sopers Lane, and the Spicers of the Ward of Chepe was formed. They conducted their business across shops and stalls selling spices, medicinal drugs and perfumes. A good deal of these men were Italian or German in origin.

Various-use herb bottles including horehound, rhubarb tincture and peppermint flavouring. (*Emma Kay*)

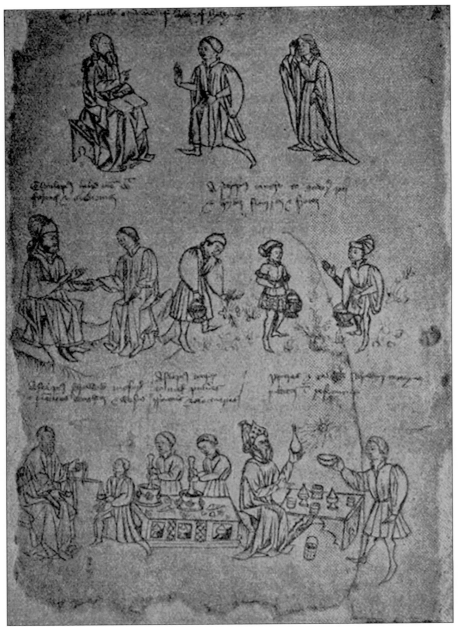

Treatises of fistula in ano, hæmorrhoids, and clysters by John Arderne, from an early fifteenth-century manuscript translation. Ed., with introduction, notes, etc., by D'Arcy Power. (*Wellcome Collection*)

Many cities and larger towns had districts dedicated to spiceries or apothecaria who traded in the local market places. A record from the City of Oxford dated 1297 mentions a district specifically housing commercial apothecaries and spicers, known as the 'Spicery'. They had market stalls in the parish of St. Mary, before moving into the parish of All Saints. There are records citing an 'Apothecaries Row' in this same parish, dated 1332.

By 1428, the rich mix of pepperers, spicers and apothecaries had merged into the Company of Grocers, officially granted charter by King Henry VI.

There are numerous references to malpractice and adulterated drugs, particularly around the fourteenth and fifteenth centuries, which led to punishments including fines, the destruction of the accused apothecary's wares and even prison.

The writings of the sixteenth-century physician, William Bullein satirically encapsulates that

He must fyrst serve God, forsee the end, be clenly, pity the poor.

Must not be suborned for money to hurt mankynde.

His place of dwelling and shop to be clenly, to please the sences withal.

His garden must be at hand with plenty of herbs, seeds, and roots.

To sow and gather, preserve and kepe them in due tyme.

To read Dioscorides, to know the nature of plants and herbes.

To invent medicines, to choose by coloure, tast, odour, figure, etc.

To have his morrters, stilles, pottes, filters, glasses, boxes, cleane and sweete.

To have charcoles at hand to make decoctions, syrupes, etc.

To keep his cleane ware closse and cast away the baggage.

To have two places in his shop, one most cleane for the physik and and a baser place for the chirurgie stuff.

That he neither increase or diminish the phisician's bill and kepe it for his own discharge.

That he neither buy nor sell rotten drugges.

That he peruse often his wares that they corrupt not.

That he put not 'quid pro quo' without advysement.

That he may open wel a vein for to help pleuresy.

That he meddle only with his vocation.
That he delyte to reede Nicholaus Myrepsus, Valerius Cordus,
Johannes Placaton, the Lubik, etc.
That he do remember that his office is only to be ye physician's cooke.
That he use true measure and weight.
And lastly-To remember his end and the judgement of God, and
thus I do commend him to God if he be not covetous or
crafty, seeking his own lucre before other men's help, succour
and comfort.[5]

Whilst it would be impossible to capture the stories of every individual British herbalist in history, this part of the chapter attempts to provide a snapshot of the lives of some of the most influential and lesser-known characters, from the academic to the pseudo. The overall narrative is also one that only extends to the beginning of the twentieth-century as by the onset of the Second World War it could be interpreted that people's conviction in the benefits of herbalism had begun to decline. Although it is fair to say that independent traders were still very much present on the streets of Britain, from 'botany shops' and certified dispensers, claiming to be members of this society or that association. Under wartime conditions there was also an acute shortage of herbs and those more traditional healers who once gathered their plants from the fields and forests were called up for military service. Together, with the inception of the National Health Service, this would mark the beginning of the end of the wise women, the village sages, simplers and local cunnings.

Although the 'simplers' and herb gatherers of old were disappearing, many hours spent scrolling through documented incidents of malpractice, as well as successful case studies, reveals an historic deep-seated anxiety and reluctance by a broad cross-section of people to place their faith in modern science, hospitals and qualified physicians, well into the twentieth century. Despite hundreds of years of scientific advancement, a significant market for alternative medicine continued to thrive in society while mistrust and fear of the wider medical communities and pharmaceutical industries prevailed. According to the British Herbalists' Union, which held its first annual meeting in Leeds in 1943, Yorkshire miners were big believers in herbal remedies, opposed to 'doctor's stuff I' bottles'. Interestingly, by the middle of the twentieth century, a quarter of all the

500 or so members of the union were based in Yorkshire and Lancashire. With one newspaper quoting: 'in the back streets of Bradford, the housing estates of Huddersfield and among the war-workers in most towns the demand for senna pods, for blood mixtures and herbal cough cures increases weekly.'[6] One of the aspects of my research that surprised me most when writing this book, was the extent with which alternative medicine was still widely being received during the nineteenth century, at a time when the application of modern medicine was well underway. In Ireland, the last instance of a crime involving witchcraft and where the law had to intervene, was as recent as 1895, in Ballyvadlea, Tipperary.[7]

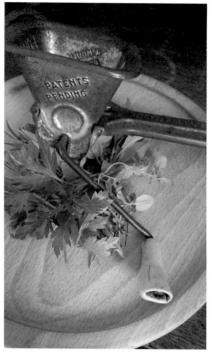

1940s 'parsmint', or herb shredder. (*Emma Kay*)

By the beginning of the twentieth century certified organizations and new regulations were also permanently changing the course of herbalism. This included the National Institute of Medical Herbalists, which was founded in the latter half of the nineteenth century, and the Society of Herbalists, in 1927, known today as The Herb Society. Key legislation extinguished the flames of ancient potions and plant lore, including the 1933 Pharmacy and Poisons Act and the Pharmacy and the Medicines Bill, of 1941 which sought to 'prohibit certain advertisements relating to medical matters and to amend the law relating to medicines'.[8]

In 1931, after many years spent researching and experimenting with plants, herbalist and author Maud Grieve introduced her long-awaited medicinal reboot, *A Modern Herbal*. This became the first comprehensive encyclopaedia of herbs to be published in English since the 1600s. It included the modern use of standardized plant extracts, reviving the herb industry for a whole new generation.

By the 1950s the frenzied advertisements of the century before, along with the public accusations of quackery significantly reduced and the old anti-witchcraft law was finally repealed in 1951. Britain's herbal narrative continues to expand and regenerate in the twenty-first century, which is fuel for at least another book or two.

Herbalists of the Fourteenth to Seventeenth Centuries

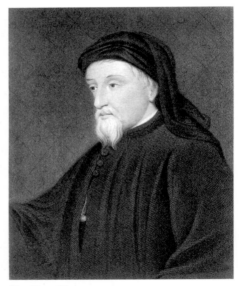

Geoffrey Chaucer.

Although he wasn't a herbalist, I'm going to open this section with a homage to the great fourteenth-century poet, Geoffrey Chaucer. Chaucer has been identified by his biographers as a bit of a botanist, as well as an author. He is one of the few writers of his time who lived alongside and directly wrote about real characters of the early medieval era.

His fictional Doctor of Physic is one of the most knowledgeable of all the characters presented in the infamous *Canterbury Tales*. He is also one of the most ruthlessly aspirational and avaricious characters. Given that his position in society is so important and respected, the Doctor of Physic is perhaps a reflection of the importance of early medics, medics who benefitted from the sick, claiming to have studied medical literature and the works of classical philosophers, when in reality they often depended on superstition and dishonest practices. David Wright is a contemporary translator of medieval works and his interpretation of the Physician in Chaucer's *Prologue* to the *Canterbury Tales* summarises everything that was untrustworthy, egotistical, and immoral about early medicine:

> With us there was a doctor, a Physician;
> Nowhere in all the world was one to match him
> Where medicine was concerned, or surgery;

Being well grounded in astrology
He'd watch his patient with the utmost care
Until he'd found a favourable hour,
By means of astrology, to give treatment.
Skilled to pick out the astrologic moment
For charms and talismans to aid the patient,
He knew the cause of every malady,
If it were 'hot' or 'cold' or 'moist' or 'dry',
And where it came from, and from which humour.
He was a really fine practitioner.
Knowing the cause, and having found its root,
He'd soon give the sick man an antidote.
Ever at hand he had apothecaries
To send him syrups, drugs, and remedies,
For each put money in the other's pocket-
Theirs was no newly founded partnership.
Well read was he in Aesculapius,
In Dioscorides, and in Rufus,
Ancient Hippocrates, hali, and galen,
Avicenna, Rhazes, and Serapion,
Averroes, Damascenus, Constantine,
Bernard, and Gilbertus,and gaddesden.
In his own diet he was temperate,
For it was nothing if not moderate,
Though most nutritious and digestible.
He didn't do much reading in the bible.
He was dressed all in Persian blue and scarlet
Lined with taffeta and fine sarsenet,
And yet was very chary of expense.
He put by all he earned from pestilence;
In medicine gold is the best cordial.
So it was gold that he loved best of all.[9]

Living and working around the same period as Chaucer, Henry Daniel was a Dominican friar and a man who was skilled in medicines and the healing arts. He maintained a garden in Stepney, London with over two-hundred varieties of plants and wrote among other literary works, an encyclopaedic manuscript of herbs along with a guide to their medicinal properties. Two different versions can be found in the British Library. Daniel also practised uroscopy, which was an early form of examining a person's urine for abnormalities. He worked in East Anglia, Stamford, and Lincoln as well as briefly in Kent and Bristol. He spent seven years studying herbs and was formally tutored, while his uroscopy skills were self-taught. He joined the Dominican Order when he found himself in dire poverty.[10]

Henricus Anglicus, or Henry English contributed to a medical treatise in the thirteenth or fourteenth century, maybe earlier, which only survives in part, but was widely cited by the herbalist Henry Daniel. Some even allege that they were one and the same person. Henricus, constructed a square herbarium and listed what and how he planted his herbs. This, in accordance with other documented square herb gardens of the Middle Ages, would have been walled or fenced, containing a central lawned area which may have included a pool or a fountain. The tallest of the plants were planted around the wall/fence, with the smallest plants edging the borders surrounding the square lawn. Henry Daniel translated the list of herbs that Henricus planted including Anglica Costus, or Costmary, which was originally used in brewing instead of hops. Aristologia, or Birthwort, a herb known to be useful in childbirth. Then there was Betha Minor, or 'a lesser beet', pennyroyal, saffron crocus, used as an opioid for pain relief and as a natural dye. Daniel also mentions Dittany from Crete, an ancient medicinal herb known for its gastric benefits. It was also one of the original ingredients of the Benedictine liqueur made in the medieval monasteries of the Trappistine and Benedictine monks. Henry actively grew white hellebore, fenugreek, violets, knotwort, lavender, myrtle, nettles, wild thyme, clary, agnus castus and hollyhock, among others.[11] Henry Daniel wrote a major herbal dubbed, *Aaron* or *Aaron Danielis*. It is a treatise that survives in one complete and one partial manuscript, held in the British Library.

William Turner of Northumberland, was one of the first English medieval botanists; a plant scientist, opposed to healer, who gained his knowledge from travelling and studying throughout Europe in the 1500s. One of his most famous works, *Libellus de re herbaria novus*, provides the first record of the specific location of British plants, along with his three-volume *Herball* which was in part dedicated to Queen

Elizabeth I. In the latter he lists the benefits of garden mint to include mitigating round worms, earache and smoothing a rough tongue.[12] Prior to travelling around England preaching the Reformation, causing chaos with the authorities and finding himself imprisoned, Turner studied at Cambridge, where he was made a fellow and then a church deacon. It was his old college who raised the funds to have Turner released. He then began his extensive travels and was granted an MD. before returning to England to marry and indulge in his love of natural history.[13]

One of the medieval period's most recognized herbalists and a trained barber-surgeon was Cheshire-born John Gerard, who managed the gardens of chief adviser to Queen Elizabeth I and patron of alchemy, Lord Burghley (William Cecil).

Some strands of medieval European alchemy endorsed the use of herbal medicines and plant remedies. Royal Principal Secretary and Lord Treasurer to Queen Elizabeth I, Lord Burghley was also an alchemist, the art of which he wove into his ministerial responsibilities.

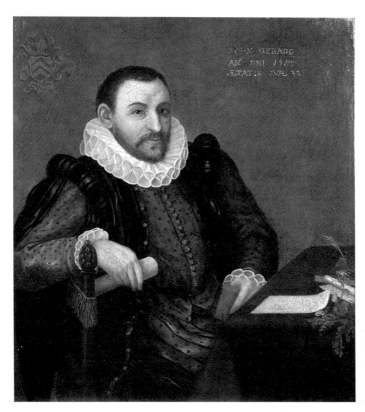

A man designated as John Gerard, Surgeon and Herbalist. (*Wellcome Collection L0001746*)

At a time when John Gerard was moving in these royal social circles, Queen Elizabeth was treated to a speech all about herbs during a visit to Sudeley Castle in 1592. The speech was documented thus:

> Herbs, maladies and stones, all maladies have cured;
> Herbs, words, and stones, I used when I loved;
> Herbs, smells, words, wind, stones hardness have procured;
> By stones, nor words, nor herbs, her mind was moved.
> I ask'd the cause: this was a woman's reason,
> 'Mongst herbs are weeds, and thereby are refused;
> Deceit, as well as Truth, speaks words in season,
> False stones by foiles have many one abused.
> I sigh'd, and then she said my fancy smoked;
> I gaz'd, she said my looks were Folly's glancing;
> I sounded dead, she said my love was choked;
> I started up, she said my thoughts were dancing.
> O, sacred Love! If thou have any Godhead,
> Teach other rules to win a maidenhead.[14]

Incidentally, Katherine Parr used an evergreen shrub called green santolina growing in the herb garden at Sudeley Castle, to ease the pains in Henry VIII's legs.[15]

Gerard was not university trained, like Turner, nor did he write or preach about God in relation to his work, as so many of his peers and contemporaries did. In 1596, he published a list of all the plants he grew in his own garden at Holborn, London. *Catalogus arborum*. Gerard's greatest work was *The Herball or General Historie of Plants*, completed in 1597. He remains a popular yet controversial figure, partly for his relentless and unfounded belief in things like trees that grew geese and seashells and for his blatant plagiarism.[16] Gerard had a knack for exaggerating his talents and embellishing the truth; ironically, his reputation has been more long-lasting than many other herbalists and botanists of his generation.

In his 1597 edition of *The Herball* something extraordinary occurs under the 'virtues' of Water Docks or Bastard Rhubarb, with John Gerard noting:

The rootes sliced and boiled in the water of Carduus Benedictus to the consumption of the third part, adding thereto a little honie, of the which decoction eight or ten sponfuls drunke before the fit, cureth the ague in two or three times of taking it at the most: vnto robustous or strong bodies, twelve sponfuls may be given. This experiment was practised by a worshipful gentlewoman called mistress Anne Wylbraham, upon divers [various] of hir poore neighbours with good success.

By including Anne in this way, Gerard legitimized her authority as a herbalist and physician, long before women were recognized as such. Clearly, she is no 'witch'. Anne is a 'gentlewoman' and a learned, charitable one at that. I can find very little information on Anne, but clearly, she was well acquainted with Gerard and very respected in her work.

We learn about another Anne acquainted with Gerard, from the journals of Lady Anne Clifford herself, whose mother Margaret Clifford, Countess of Cumberland, was 'deeply interested in alchemy and she found out many excellent medicines that did good to many people and that she distilled waters and chemical extractions, delighting in the work'. Lady Anne herself was a known admirer of the herbalist John Gerard, with one of the family portraits depicting his work in the background.

Women's interest in herbalism and botany it seems was a widespread occupation. Margaret Boscawen's 'plant notebook' is a surviving written example of medicinal plants from the seventeenth century. Her twelve-page notebook discusses plants, flowers, roots and seeds with details about drying and distilling. Most interesting was Boscawen's source of irritation at not being able to freely access the herbs and plants she needed from her own locality. She talks about having to send to London for items including horseradish, gentian, citron and the bark of the black alder tree. She may well have been able to acquire these locally but chose instead to obtain them from London, based perhaps on the fact that she took most of her information from Culpeper, who lists where specifically to source these items in London.[18]

In former, bleaker times women were not allowed to own their own property, but widows who were considered to be competent, were granted permission to continue running a family business in the absence of a husband. The archives provide evidence of women working as apothecaries under these circumstances. The 'Widow Wynke', wife of Tobias Wynke, was allocated £2 annually by the Company of Apothecaries, from 1628 onwards. She became an independent apothecary and ran her own shop. She was even granted an apprentice. Apprentices were well known for being difficult to manage. The work and hours were long and arduous and it took seven years to become fully trained. Widow Wynke's first apprentice was accused of physically and verbally abusing his employer. She must have had some clout to persuade the Company of Apothecaries to let the young man

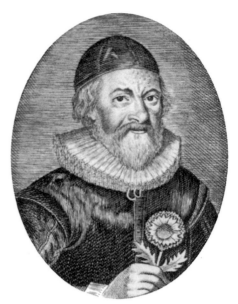

John Parkinson.

go on these terms, providing her with the opportunity to garner a new assistant. Often the legacies of the husbands of these women and the respect they were honoured in life, transferred to the widows.[19]

John Gerard's peer, John Parkinson, born around 1567, was apothecary to James I and Royal Botanist to Charles I. His 1629 publication, *Paradisi in Sole Paradisus Terrestris* (Park-In Sun's *Terrestil Paradise*), was a pun of his name. He placed himself in the centre of his own garden of paradise.

Parkinson kept his botanical garden in London's Covent Garden which may have exceeded two acres. His celebrated bestseller, *Theatrum Botanicum* (*Theatre of Plants*), was published in 1640 and was Parkinson's most significant work.[20] But Parkinson's origins were humble, from a long line of Lancashire farmworkers, but by the time John's father James died, he had managed to acquire some considerable wealth, including several farms, the lease to a corn mill and a blacksmith's. Growing up in a wild and fertile landscape between the Ribble and Calder valleys, somewhere in the region of Bleasdale and Whalley, John and his siblings would have roamed free to enjoy everything the area offered, with the surrounding moors providing some of the food to be gathered to accompany their meals. As a much older man, Parkinson would reminisce:

If I should set down all sortes of herbes that are usually gathered for sallets I should not only speak of Garden herbes, but of many … that grow wild in the fields, or else be but weeds in a garden. For the usual manner of many is to take the young buds and leaves of everything almost that growth. As well in the garden as in the Fields, and put them all together, that the taste of the one may amend the relish of the other.[21]

Throughout his life, Parkinson was committed to herbs as strengthening and nourishing additions to food and as medicinal aids:

The former age of our great Grandfathers, had all these hot herbes in much and familiar use, both for their meates and medicines, and therewith preserved themselves in long life and much health: but this delicate age of ours, which is not pleased with anything almost, be it meat or medicine, that is not pleasant to the palate, does wholly refuse these almost, and therefore cannot be partaker of the benefit of them.[22]

The other great love of his life, Catholicism, forced John Parkinson to live forever in the shadow of the Reformation; it split his family apart and resulted in him leaving the Church for good in 1603.[23]

Descendant and author of Parkinson's most recent biography at the time of writing, Anna Parkinson, summarizes his character, as simply, 'The man of the soil'. [24]

And so, to a name that has sustained most recognition, if only for his popular household manual, the *Complete Herbal*. A bit like Mrs Beeton's book of *Household Management*, Nicholas Culpeper's comprehensive reference book of herbs is one that could be found in many a home, right into the twentieth century.

Born into the Stuart era, when much of the population of Britain was sheltering against a backdrop of poverty, high levels of mortality, political unrest, inequality and mistrust, others basked in the benefits of extensive trading in the global marketplace, with greater accessibility to luxury goods, business opportunities and a surge of interest in the arts. Culpeper, whose surname actually means 'mischief maker', was fascinated by the world of astronomy and astrology and the myriad of medicinal plants introduced to him as a child. Raised by his mother and a grandfather whom he both feared and disrespected, Nicholas found solace in the maternal world of food, household chores, healing and nurturing. He worshipped his mother Mary who, having experienced so much sickness and death in her young life, learnt to treat wounds and mix medicines aplenty. It became young Nicholas's job to go and retrieve the necessary plants required for these medicines from the fertile and magical landscape that circled Ashdown Forest. But his grandfather had other plans for him and at age 10, Nicholas was packed off to grammar school, before extending his education in theology at Cambridge University in 1632 – a career move imposed on him by his grandfather.

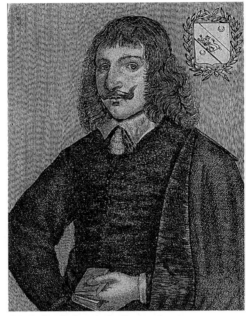

Nicholas Culpeper by Richard Gaywood.

While at Cambridge Nicholas met the girl he wanted to marry, Judith. Anticipating his grandfather's disapproving reaction, they planned to elope. During the journey to their union, his bride-to-be died of shock travelling through a thunderstorm. Heartbroken and distraught, Nicholas deserted Cambridge and his family home in Sussex. His new home and life became opportunist London.[25]

Biographers of Culpeper differ in their outlook during this phase of his life. Some say it was his grandfather who forced him to move away and repent his sins, to make a career as an apothecary; others that Nicholas just continued to rebel. He had after all, always had a keen interest in herbal medicine. In 1634 he became an apprentice within the Apothecaries Society and went through several masters for a variety of reasons, none to do with Culpeper personally. Apprentices were exploited, abused and mistreated in the 1600s and there was no legislation to dictate anything otherwise. As a young man making his way in the big, challenging capital Culpeper was documented by friends and colleagues as having both a wicked sense of humour and an irritable temper.

Apothecaries were expressly forbidden to practise medicine, but that did not stop Culpeper or his best friend Samuel Leadbetter. Apothecaries were trained simply to mix medicines, not to dispense them. But, during the seventeenth century in England, more and more apothecaries were shifting their roles. So, while we could accuse Culpeper of illegal quackery, we must also recognize that countless others were following suit and by the time of the Great Plague, many people would willingly open their arms to be treated by apothecaries, as physicians dropped like flies in the wake of that cruel pandemic.

Culpeper frowned upon exotic medicines like opium and senna. He liked working with simple, common herbs and respected ancient, traditional remedies over new concoctions. He rarely strayed from the philosophies of Galen and dismissed herbs from overseas, not because they were foreign, but because he believed they would not suit the constitutions of English people. Culpeper criticized physicians who focused on the disease, rather than studying the patient and loathed the practice of diagnosis by analysing a patient's urine, which was a common practice then. Nicholas focused on the wellbeing of the person as a whole, including all aspects of their demeanour, checking their eyes, ears, nose, the odour of their breath, spit and faeces. He also used astrological charts, but his processes of diagnosis and treatment were rational and considered in their approach. He built himself a reputation as a good healer in London within a short space of time. Wealthy grain merchant Charles Field suffered greatly with a type of gout, which no one seemed able to ease. As a rising new medic in the area, Culpeper was sent for. He did what no other physic could and, in the process, ended up marrying Field's daughter, Alice. They would go on to have seven children together, although many died at a young age.[26]

Ever the rebel and anti-authoritarian, Culpeper fought on the side of the Parliamentarians during the English Civil War, translated many medical texts from Latin to English to make them more accessible to the general public, condemned greed, exposed charlatan practices and discredited the commercialization of medicine. Culpeper's methods were strange but they often worked with effect. Undeniably he has one of the strongest legacies of all the herbalists of his age, and rightly so.

Late medieval herbalists lived in times of great transition. Advancements in printing and publishing were revolutionizing access to knowledge.

Communication, global exploration and burgeoning foreign trade were altering the cultural and economic landscape of Britain. Yet, many aspects of medieval life remained shrouded in superstition, ignorance and poverty. Nuns and early midwives aside, there are few recorded early British female herbalists, possibly due to the fact that for centuries they were stigmatized as fiendish, and women were unlikely to be published unless they were noble or monied. Witchcraft was undoubtedly a notion perpetuated by Christians to hamper the spread of knowledge – both good and potentially evil. Throw in some early medieval misogyny and male-dominated jurisdiction and the Witchcraft Act of 1542 was created, prescribing the death penalty for any crimes involving invocations, conjuring and spells. This legislation changed over the years, from being repealed to replaced, with more specific laws imposed relating to the conjuring up of evil spirits or committing murder through magic.

The Anglo-Saxon abbess, Hilda of Whitby, was born a noblewoman and according to Bede:

'The Island of the Hart', at that time ruled by the Abbess Hilda, who, two years after, having acquired an estate of ten families, at the place called Streanaeshalch, built a monastery there, in which the aforesaid king's daughter was first trained in the monastic life and afterwards became abbess; till, at the age of fifty-nine, the blessed virgin departed to be united to her Heavenly Bridegroom.[27]

Author Elisabeth Brooke confirmed that Hilda taught and practised medicine most of her life, as well as being a skilled healer.[28] She is one of the first to be recorded as such.

As outlined in the introduction, midwifery, which was the main form of physic for women during the early medieval period, was held in suspicion during the 1500s. The Church became responsible in England for regulating these practices, with midwives having to swear oaths to God that any stillborn births would receive a secret burial, far away from supernatural influences. Midwives were also forbidden to utter any charms or medicate using herbs.

You shall not in any way wise use or exercise any manner of witchcraft, charm or sorcery, invocation or other prayers that may stand with god's laws and the king's. You should not give any counsel or minister any herb, medicine or potion, or any other thing, to any woman being with child whereby she should destroy or cast out that she goeth withal before her time.

By the 1700s this oath also came with a fee of up to eighteen shillings, in lieu of a paid licence to practise.[29]

Elizabeth Hales, a midwife from London, was accused of causing a woman to become delirious after administering 'long pepper and graynes in burnt wine' in 1631. Joan Ramsey, also a midwife, confessed to killing one of her patients in 1630, by dispensing bryony roots in white wine, causing the recipient to vomit, purge and die. Hales got off with a warning, while Ramsey was 'forgiven', which may indicate a relaxing of laws relating to midwives at this time in England.[30]

There were numerous 'white witches' that roamed the medieval English countryside, applying herbal remedies, simple charms and divinatory ways of healing, predicting and protecting but there were those who practised the black arts for disreputable ends. But these were few and far between. Many, like Erskine of Dun, who was beheaded along with his three sisters in 1613 for using poisonous herbs obtained from a supposed

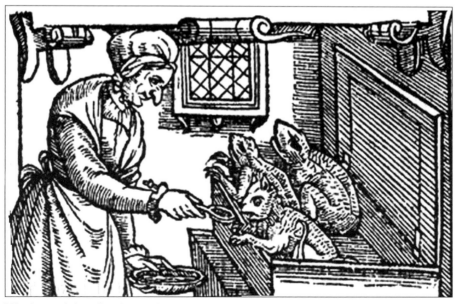

Witches and their familiars, 1579.

witch to kill their two nephews and acquire inherited wealth, made use of these maleficent resources.[31] Despite the supernatural connotations, old wise women were often respected in communities and their knowledge revered. Herbalists, including John Skelton and Americans Samuel Thomson and Albert Coffin, all learnt their trades from these wise sages. In fact, most women used herbs on a daily basis as part of their regular household duties.

Elizabeth Jackson, an elderly lady, was serving time in prison at the turn of the seventeenth century, imprisoned for casting magic spells over a sick young girl called Mary Glover, whose disease turned out to be natural and not possession by the devil. Ten members of Elizabeth's local community came forward to speak of her good character and after further investigation the old woman was finally found innocent three years later.[32]

Like many women of the seventeenth century, diarist Elizabeth Freke collected medicinal remedies and her vast collection provides tremendous insight into household medicines of the day. Born in Wiltshire, but dividing her time between England and Ireland, before settling in Norfolk, Elizabeth had close contact with a number of medical practitioners throughout her life; she made up numerous medicines and specialist 'waters' which she kept in her cupboards to cover a multitude of ailments. There is a common thread that runs throughout the virtues

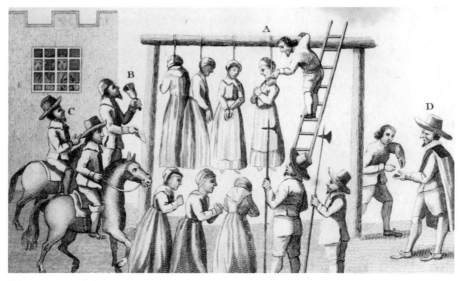

Women hanged for witchcraft, Newcastle, 1655.

of the plants she lists, namely, angelica, baume, saffron and nutmeg for feelings of bloating and general stomach disorders; saffron, ivy, nutmeg and rosemary for liver complaints; saffron and poppy for coughs and lung disorders; scurvy grass and lemon water for facial blemishes; angelica and gillyflower for fevers; baume, angelica and gillyflower for heart conditions; and for head issues relating to the brain, rosemary and nutmeg.[33]

It would be remiss not to give mention here to two rather overlooked English plant specialists who also contributed to the overall dialogue of herbology during this era: John Ray and anatomist Nehemiah Grew. John Ray or Wray was from Essex, a Cambridge graduate and fellow of the Royal Society. He travelled extensively documenting flora and fauna, both in Britain and throughout Europe and was widely published. In his 1677 *Catalogue Plantarum Angliae*, Ray included a huge list of herbs together with their appropriate prescription. He was a pragmatic man, disinterested in astrology or alchemy. His work was scientific and based on observation and experimentation. The botanist and founder of the Linnean Society, which is dedicated to the study of natural history, Sir James Smith, said of Ray: 'Our immortal naturalist, the most accurate in observation, the most philosophical in contemplation, and the most faithful in description of all the botanists of his own or perhaps and other time.'[34] Ray's legacy includes several societies and charities dedicated to raising awareness of the natural environment.

Nehemiah Grew's great work of 1680, *The Anatomy of Plants*, was born out of a series of short pamphlets he wrote about botany over a ten-year period. Although his work appears to have slipped into obscurity, Grew was one of the first to integrate microscope studies of plant morphology which led to a pioneering understanding of the internal structure of plants and the establishment of modern botany. His research contributed considerably to the broader scientific discourse of chemistry, his greatest discovery probably being that of Epsom salts.[35]

The way in which the study of herbs and plants has evolved, is characteristic of British society's transformation into a burgeoning enlightened state, where plants transposed from ritual objects to items of scientific importance over a 300-year period.

Herbalists of the Eighteenth and Nineteenth Centuries

Botanist John Hill was discredited as a consequence of numerous grudges he made public throughout the mid-eighteenth century, which undoubtedly tainted the longevity of his reputation and place within the general order of influential herbalists and botanists. Having crossed swords with the Royal Society and various other peers, Hill launched a series of literary battles against everyone he took umbrage with. His *Useful Family Herbal* of 1755, which is actually incredibly thorough, was reprinted numerous times and Hill was known to have practised herbal medicine illegally to boost his funds. He remains an excellent example of all that was good and bad about life in Georgian London; in today's poisonous social media marketplace, Hill probably would have thrived.[36] He was identified as a bit of a witch himself for practising his quackery, along with countless other names in the field of botany and herbology, who straddled the two worlds of dark arts and scholastic enrichment. 'Witches' were most certainly not always women. James Murrell was known as 'Cunning Murrell', cunning being another name for professional folk magicians, or 'white witches'. He was born in Rochford, Essex in 1781 and he went to work in London as a chemist's assistant, before returning to Essex in 1810 and trying his hand at shoemaking, a business that left him bankrupt. But James had also started to put all the knowledge he had acquired in London into practice – most notably with counteracting spells. In 1867, local historian Philip Benton wrote of Murrell:

> He supplemented his subsistence by telling fortunes [and as] a herbalist, administered potions and drugs. He would purchase forty different nostrums at a time, his price being one penny for each, which he refused to have labelled. A sack full of letters were destroyed at his death, but enough remained to prove that an amount of ignorance, credulity, superstition existed, which appears incredible. Some addressed to him allude to the appearance of apparitions, and from the tenor of others from women, mysteriously alluding to being in trouble, and hearing that he could relieve them, we may suspect him of dark doings.

Despite Benton's damning characterization, it is apparent from other records, including those noted by the local vicar, that Murrell was a well-respected man locally, particularly with the farmworkers. As well as general healer he became a skilled animal doctor, astrologer and matchmaker – a valued member of the community. James roamed Daws Heath collecting his herbs and plants and his house was said to be filled with all manner of botanical flora and fauna. His 'witch bottles' were notorious, hand-forged by a blacksmith from Hadleigh and filled with blood, water, fingernails, hair, urine and other potent ingredients. He used these to combat the effects of the dark arts, by removing spells and reversing charms.[37]

Timothy Crowther was a parish clerk from Skipton, Yorkshire, who lived from 1694 to 1761 and managed to successfully carry on trading as a cunning man alongside his more outwardly respectable position in society. One of Crowther's final acts was to find a missing man. Allegedly (and somewhat dubiously), he achieved this by having a young boy stare into a mirror until the missing man's murder was somehow reflected in the glass. He mainly dealt in cases of bewitchment and the recovery of lost goods. Crowther's legacy is his charm book which was discovered in a bookstore about 100 years after his death, containing ceremonial incantations and a myriad of spells mostly lifted from the text of *The Lesser Key of Solomon*, a famous grimoire of the Renaissance period.[38]

By reclassifying an illness or an ailment as witchcraft, cunning men and women were given licence by their communities to treat people by magical means and while some may have found success, others more often than not proved ineffectual. Norfolk stone dresser and cunning man on the side, James Stagg emphasized during his trial in 1877 that members of the community approached him when they had given up on their doctors. He attempted to cure a labourer's daughter by applying a 'peculiar looking leaf on her hand', while chanting an incantation. The treatment failed and the girl died several weeks later.[39]

Other keen herbalists dabbled less in magic and more in the tried and tested evidence behind the healing properties of nature. Born in Kendal in 1694, Dr Richard Shepherd settled in Preston around the age of 30, as a physician, bequeathing his library of thousands of volumes to the city, following his death in 1761. Shepherd lived on a property near the King's Head Inn, Friargate, which has long since disappeared, but in the gardens at the rear he cultivated angelica for medicinal purposes, which he gave away to the poorer communities of the city. During Shepherd's lifetime, angelica was highly prized for its wide variety of medicinal attributes, more of which you can read about in the next chapter. Many of the books Shepherd bequeathed to the city had a strong medical content.

He was of considerable standing in the community and sat in office as the mayor's bailiff, before being elected an alderman in 1746 and mayor in 1747, taking a second office in 1755. He and his wife Margaret, née Appleton, inherited Little Merlay Hall near Clitheroe, from her father. Built in the late sixteenth century, the property has survived as a Grade II-listed building which can still be seen today.[40] Much of Shepherd's collection of books were medical, including a book on anatomy by Felix Platter, dated 1583, and an anatomical atlas with to-scale drawings.[41] He is buried in the grounds of St. George's Church on Lune Street, Preston. His library of books which formed the foundation of Preston's Harris Museum is not the only legacy he left behind: his collection was first housed in a building located on Shepherd Street. (You can find a recipe for angelica pie, from Burnley, Lancashire, in Chapter 3.)

Elizabeth Blackwell, née Blachrie, came from a wealthy Aberdeen-based family and is best known for her illustrations, along with her

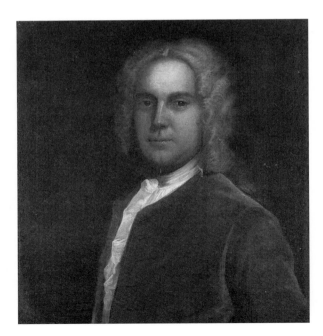

Dr Richard Shepherd, by Hamlet Winstanley, oil on canvas, about 1735. (*Harris Museum, Art Gallery & Library, Preston*)

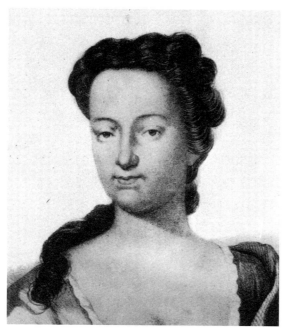

Elizabeth Blackwell.

one published medicinal reference book titled, *A Curious Herbal*. Born around 1707, as a young girl she eloped with her second cousin, a medical student called Alexander Blackwell, before the couple moved to London. Elizabeth began training as a midwife to assist her husband in his practice, but abandoned this later in life. Alexander also abandoned his medical calling and attempted to establish himself as a printer. Not being fully trained in this profession, he was not taken seriously and quickly fell into debt for which he was committed to prison for two years.

Elizabeth's talents as an amateur artist and botanist, which she gained from her excellent education growing up in Aberdeen, provided her with the motivation to earn the funds to repay her husband's debts and release him from prison.[42]

She was guided in part by Sir Hans Sloane and Dr Richard Mead who encouraged her in her work. She also took lodgings adjacent to Chelsea Physic Garden, so that she was best placed to study her subject in detail. It took years to draw the plants by hand, engrave them and colour them, as well as engraving the text itself. She published her work as a series of weekly editions between 1737 and 1739. The College of Physicians 'so greatly approved of it that they not only made her a handsome present, but also gave her ample testimonial, in writing, of their approbation of her work'.[43.]

Her published studies were overall a great success and Elizabeth was able to release Alexander from prison. Having started and left another job in London under a discredited cloud, Alexander took up a post with the ambassador to Sweden, leaving Elizabeth alone in London with a young child. Alexander called himself a physick and was appointed to treat King Frederick, but was quickly exposed as a quack and so took up another post in agriculture,

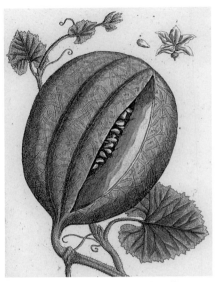

Illustration by Elizabeth Blackwell.

which he also managed to botch. Desperate to reinstate himself in society, Alexander is alleged to have participated in a plot to place the Duke of Cumberland on the Swedish throne, but was found guilty of treason before being arrested, tortured and beheaded. Elizabeth was due to follow her husband to Sweden and it is not known what happened to her next. All three of her children died young. It is estimated she died around 1758 and is buried in London.[44]

Less educated and refined, Amelia Woodcock was known locally as 'The Wise Woman of Wing', Wing being a village near the market town of Uppingham in Rutland. She had no formal medical training but her reputation for treating all manner of illnesses, including cancer, was known throughout the area. In her early years of practising healing Amelia spent a great deal of time gathering herbs from local fields and woods, but as soon as she started gaining more clients and notoriety, she abandoned the woods and ordered what she needed from the local chemist. People of all classes, including qualified physicians, would visit her little cottage daily, either for advice or to be treated. She often had so many customers that visitors took to staying overnight in the village itself or neighbouring locations. Her concoctions were not overpowering or dangerous, but she did have a reputation for providing generous doses for her clients to take away with them. It was also said she was gifted in some sort of ability to diagnose on sight.

A newspaper of the time, acquired some of her letters sent to a chemist who regularly supplied her with drugs and published them:

Sir will you send Mrs woodcock 1 galland of savalatta, 1 of red lavender 3 of niter 7 pound of jelap and 7 iripica half stone of juniper beries and anne seeds 6 bottles 6 bottles of quaninea small passil of red salve 1 dozen of skins and 10s worth of coft pills 2 bladders of seam 4 stone of tireacle as early as conveoien.
Atnealla Woodcook

Dear fren eye have sent you a small order if you think well to excep it 6 gallands of niter and a large bottle of dark mixture 1 galland of savaletta 1 galland of lavender 1 quart of oil of juneper and 6 pound of black plaster the same of red and 3 pound of gelap 3 of hilepica 6 bottles of quine.

Iripica, which she also calls hilepica, was a favourite of Amelia's and was said to be a mixture brought back from Jamaica, the contents of which she never divulged.

Amelia died quite young in the 1860s, before she reached middle age, from lack of exercise, as it was widely reported that she rarely left the house.[45]

Amelia's story legitimizes the existence and popularity of traditional herbal medicine well into the Victorian age, but by the 1700s the study of plant life as a science was evolving and with it a new breed of botanical experts. Sir Hans Sloane was an illustrious British physician and botanist who straddled the seventeenth and eighteenth centuries. Born in Ireland, his medical training was taken up in London and overseas, while he mastered the art of botany at the Chelsea Physic Garden. He became a physician at Christ's Hospital early in his career and succeeded Sir Isaac Newton as president of the Royal Society in 1712. Sloane was made a baronet four years later and then took the position of George II's physician in 1727. He travelled extensively throughout Jamaica recording and accumulating a wealth of botanical material, material which formed several journals, but he only published one work: *An Account of a Medicine for Soreness, Weakness, and Other Distempers of the Eyes*. Despite the glowing credentials, Sloane has faced a great deal of criticism, in life and in death, as someone who knew how to manipulate the right people and move in influential circles. His contributions to science were limited. His wealth and collections, largely gained from the profits of slavery, helped establish the foundations of London's British Museum.[46] For inflamed eyes Sloane recommended a conserve of rosemary flowers, antiepileptic powders, betony, sage, rosemary, eyebright, wild valerian root and castor washed down with a tea made of some of the same ingredients.[47]

The antithesis to Sloane, a radical Socialist and member of the London Working Men's Association, John Skelton was a practising herbalist originally from the West Country, who relied on Thomsonian principles, created by the American self-taught botanist, Samuel Thomson. These principles were, among other things, based on the notion of purging toxins via steam treatments and homemade preparations. Skelton also advocated the use of indigenous, North American and tropical herbs.

He qualified as a medical practitioner in 1863 and was committed to the role of nature in healing, which was apparent in his 1853 publication of *A Plea for the Botanic Practice of Medicine*; he actively supported the use of herbal medicine in working-class communities.[48] Wise women were often as much credited as they were criticized or feared. John Skelton learnt his trade from an old woman, a healer and midwife, his grandmother, who took the young John with her when she went gathering herbs. She taught him how to identify plants and where to locate them, as well as instructing him on the ways in which they could be used to treat the sick of the village. Throughout his life, Skelton frequently referenced his grandmother as his teacher and greatest inspiration.

Having established his own practice, John Skelton became deputy to the notorious American MD, Albert Coffin, who managed to flee his country in the wake of a trial for murder. Coffin dispatched John up to the North of England where he soon became indispensable to him. Poverty in the north was rife throughout the Industrial age; with families living hand to mouth in tiny, crowded communities, with poor sanitation surrounded by the smog and fumes belting out from the factories. People needed ongoing medical help and Skelton was there to fill the role. After a brief departure from Coffin's leadership where Skelton moved to Edinburgh and established a new practice, he returned to his colleague's side to disseminate the theories of Coffinism throughout Wales. Realizing that Coffin was both exploiting and keeping Skelton out of the limelight, he eventually and successfully set up in competition to Albert in the North of England and became a shrewd businessman importing herbs and recruiting agents to his new practice.[49]

Traversing both the Victorian and Edwardian eras, horticulturist, botanist and writer, Alicia Margaret Tyssen Amherst was the author of England's first academic account of the history of gardening. She was privileged and well connected in society with access to diverse scholarly material, but travelled widely, including Africa, Australia and New Zealand, collecting plant samples. Amherst was instrumental in raising the profile of women working in horticulture, but her achievements have been somewhat overlooked despite leaving a legacy of several books, including her seminal work, *A History of Gardening*, published in 1895.[50] Amherst provided a unique insight into some aspects of herb gardens, informing her readers about the old custom of the 'still room', where (mostly) women would prepare and conserve fruits, distil and fashion decoctions using numerous herbs directly from the garden, recalling the long-forgotten sixteenth-century poetry of Thomas Tusser and his *Five Hundred Points of Good Husbandry*:

> Good aqua composita, vinegar tart
> Rose water and treacle to comfort the hart.
> Cold herbs in hir garden for agues that burne
> That ouer strong heat to good temper may turne.
>
> Get water of fumentoire, Liuer to coole
> And others the like, or els lie like a foole
> Conserue of the Barbarie, Quinces and such
> With sirops that easeth the sickley so much.

Amherst catalogued the cultivation of garden herbs specifically for medicinal purposes, including a list of 'herbes to stylle' recorded in a document from 1502:

Borage, columbine, buglos [borage] sorrel, cowsloppes [cowslips], scabious [from the honeysuckle family], wild tansey, wormwood, endyff [chicory], sauge [sage], dandelion and hart's tongue [an evergreen fern].[51]

She received an OBE in 1918 for her prolific work within the field of gardening and garden history.

Some readers might recognize the name of Napier as a prominent one in the world of botanical heritage. The eminent Scottish Victorian herbalist, Duncan Napier, is the man behind Napier's of Edinburgh, established in 1860 and still trading as one of the few remaining high-street herbal shops and clinics in Britain, now with stores trading in Bathgate and Glasgow.

Duncan was rejected by his biological mother at birth and was adopted by a publican. His early life was hard and he was regularly beaten by his adoptive mother. His one solace was the summer months which he spent in the countryside with the family of a regular patron of the pub. It was here that Duncan would start to learn all about nature and plants. At the age of 14 he became an apprentice baker and two years later was lucky enough to acquire a mentor, a man who introduced him to a formal education, the temperance movement, and the Church. As a baker his lungs became affected by the flour dust and so Napier experimented with lobelia, creating a syrup which relieved his cough within a matter of months. It was from hereon in that his passion for herbal remedies began. Duncan would spend hours collecting the plants he needed to experiment before finally being funded by his mentor to start trading as a herbalist.[52] His diaries acknowledge:

> During the months of April and May I used to get up very early in the morning to get my herbs, and I might have been standing in Duddingston Loch any time in the morning from four to seven o'clock, with my shoes and stockings off and trousers rolled up as far as they would go, pulling up buckbean. It was as much as I could do in those cold mornings to stand in the cold water, but I usually carried home a heavy bag full of buckbean, well up for a hundredweight, I got a good heat before I got home. It took me two days before I got each load tied into bunches and hung up to dry.[53]

Buck- or bog-bean has traditionally been equated with digestion and as a plant that can both increase the appetite and act as a laxative. More recently bog-bean has become known for its anti-inflammatory characteristics.

Duncan Napier became associated with his widely known Nerve Debility Tonic, the primary ingredient of which was oats. He developed this remedy to help the thousands of customers who requested assistance with stress and exhaustion. Not such a modern-day malady after all then![54] He married and had an extensive family whom he tutored in all that he had learnt about plants and herbs, his son Duncan II recalling:

> We had to go into the country and gather herbs for my father's business: yarrow, eyebright, comfrey, agrimony, wormwood, tansy, elder flowers, woundwort, hawthorn berries, to name only a few.[55]

His sons joined the business which was renamed D. S. Napier & Sons in 1905. The shop stayed in the family for several generations, John Napier being the last in line. During the 1990s the premises were acquired by a medical herbalist, Dee Atkinson, who restored the business along with many of the old original recipes. It continues to thrive today.

Quackery and Hazardous Herbology

By the seventeenth century some of the stalwart Greek and Roman medical doctrines started to be challenged and there was a blurring of professions, with physicians, surgeons, apothecaries and traditional herbalists often melting into one craft. 'For the doctor relies on the druggists and the druggists on a greedy and dirty old woman, with the audacity and capacity to impose anything on him'. As a consequence, the legitimacy of the physick garden became central to the study of medicine, as places where plants could be identified and studied in an official scholarly manner.[56]

While some herbalists and physicians undoubtedly had the skills to ease the pain of others, they could just as easily cause more damage than good. For every genuine healer, there were many more willing to exploit the suffering of others for their own gain. Perhaps some practitioners were more misguided than nefarious, but whatever their motives, the archives are bursting with stories of malpractice.

In 1826, Jacob Evans wrote his *British Herbal or Medicinal Book*, the same year that he was indicted for murdering a 17-year-old cabinetmaker's apprentice, Camp Collins. Having complained of dizzy spells, which impacted on his daily work, Collins's employer, John Burbidge, called on his colleague Evans, who he knew had written a book about herbal remedies, requesting his help with treating the boy. Evans's prescription was 'two or three pennyworths of fox-glove' to be boiled in water.[57] Sure enough, a couple of hours after drinking the concoction, Camp Collins fell so ill that he had to retreat to bed. He died the following morning and an autopsy concluded that the cause of death was 'vegetable poisoning'. The amount of foxglove which had been administered was twelve to fifteen times the quantity of the standard safe dose.

According to Evans's book, man was born disease free and thus sinful behaviour was the consequence of all illness. He determined that God provided the world with an abundance of herbs to alleviate any number of illnesses. Despite the boy's death and a damning report issued by the surgeon who attended to Collins while he was dying, Jacob Evans was found guilty of manslaughter, opposed to murder. Other remedies that Evans endorsed included leaves from a fig tree for leprosy and bistort (a pink flowering plant from the dock family), to cure smallpox and measles.

Dr Albert. I. Coffin, as mentioned earlier in this chapter, had a practice at 134 High Holborn, London, during the mid-1800s. He wrote prolifically on medical botany and administered all manner of compounds and elixirs. He was very well known and respected in England, with John Skelton becoming his assistant in 1848. Coffin was an American, who introduced new approaches to herbalism in England. In the 1830s and it was Coffin and Skelton who gathered trained herbalists together to form an association known later in 1864 as the National Institute of Medical Herbalists, essentially synthesizing the American Thomsonian approach with traditional European methods. The institute remains one of the oldest and largest of its kind.

At Stephen Hill, Upper Hallam, Sheffield, during an outbreak of typhus, there was an inquiry into the death of a 40-year-old woman, Hannah Finningley. Hannah was treated by a non-medical professional, William Fox, a former joiner from Bolton, Lancashire, who was a follower of Dr Coffin's theories and a former agent of his work. Fox had been practising for around ten years or so, regularly prescribing yarbs to people in the local neighbouring communities. Mrs Finningley had a raging fever and inflammation, which impacted on both her mind and body. Fox prescribed skull-cap and English and American valerians, skull-cap being known to help with problems relating to the nervous system. He also administered yarrow, hyssop and pennyroyal for her fever, combined with mixtures containing sage, rosemary, catnip, aniseeds and the milk of bitter almonds, all of which were to be taken four times a day.

Fox did not charge for his services, only for the cost of the herbs. When Hannah's health started to decline further, a medical doctor was called in by a concerned local vicar but her husband refused his suggested treatments, subsequently leading to the death of his wife.

The house and the entire neighbourhood were drowning in filth and squalor and during the inquiry into his wife's death, Hannah's husband was persuaded reluctantly to take the advice of the medical practitioner where caring for his children, who were also ill, was concerned. The final verdict was death by typhoid and William Fox was absolved of any culpability.[58]

While Fox's herbal treatments probably did not contribute to Hannah Finningley's death, they did nothing to help her either and if a trained doctor had been able to care for her, she may have at least received a more comforting death. There are thousands of similar cases recorded during the Victorian era where trained physicians came into conflict with traditional herbalists in this way. The reality was that even an educated, science-based training back in the nineteenth century did very little to cure or ease the suffering of people dying from typhoid or cholera. These were diseases born out of the filthy urban conditions of nineteenth-century society. By the very end of the century Joseph Lister's germ theory, would eventually lead to vaccinations and improved living conditions, but until then, both qualified and non-qualified medical practitioners were all working in a similar degree of ignorance.

James Wallis, whose shop premises were located at 34 Bath Street, City Road, London, fatally administered lobelia to Matilda Sainsbury in 1884. Lobelia was sometimes used as an expectorant. A professor of medicine, Dr Thomas Stevenson was brought in to investigate on behalf of the Home Office and determined that while half of the bottle prescribed would not have fatal consequences, consuming the bottle in its entirety would. Matilda only drank half of the contents, so Wallis was still considered culpable. In his statement he declared:

I sent the woman lobelia but it is a lie to say it is poison. My wife has taken double the quantity. That fool of a doctor who gave evidence yesterday knows nothing about it. The medical science of this country is a fraud. God made the world and gave herbs for everything, but doctors don't know how to use them. Lobelia is not a poison and it was struck off the list of poisons before a committee of the House of Lords in 1857.

Wallis was found innocent as it was determined there was no criminal negligence or disregard to human life. This was based on the testimonies of numerous herbalists who came forward to confirm the common use of lobelia to treat ailments successfully and without danger. The defence also confirmed that large doses administered to other patients were not known to be problematic.[59]

It's important to note that in many court cases, evidence of malpractice often came down to the dosage of a herb which could shift from medicinal to fatal in a matter of ounces. Frequently patients who were prescribed herbs in various forms did not measure according to the instructions given.

People retained faith in herbalists as they successfully cured an array of ailments. Whether it was just luck that the illness dissipated at the same time the remedy was administered, or a placebo affect was achieved, or that the restorative properties of a natural remedy genuinely mitigated symptoms. Whatever the circumstances, it was significant enough for people to continue to employ herbal practitioners. While herbalists had a proven legacy stretching thousands of years, trained doctors of science remained controversial and were treated with suspicion.

Thirty-two-year-old pregnant Eliza Wilson died after managing to give one final statement to a justice of the peace from her bed on 20 September 1848. The father of the child persuaded her to visit a herbalist. The first gave her a mixture of pills and other tinctures which failed to work. The second herbalist, Mrs Lindfield, ran a herb shop in East Street, Walworth. Lindfield used a catheter, amongst other instruments, internally on Eliza to induce a miscarriage. This procedure was carried out several times. Lindfield then prescribed Epsom salt when Eliza became ill and suggested placing her feet in warm water. It emerged during the trial that Lindfield had also administered Eliza with pills containing among other ingredients, 'five-leaved grass [and] ground ivy'. Eliza's death was attributed to:

inflammation of the bladder, the uterus, and the peritoneum; she had certainly advanced into the second month of pregnancy, abortion had taken place, and I should suppose from unnatural causes.

It was suggested during the trial that savin was also prescribed, which was frequently used to induce miscarriages, but there was no direct evidence to support this. Several women came forward to vouch for her services and character and Lindfield was found not guilty.[60]

In the nineteenth century, a whole cornucopia of drugs and herbs could be accessed from quacks to chemists, to stimulate miscarriages, including tansy and pennyroyal, quinine, and turpentine.[61] Interestingly, savin is a species of juniper and gin is made with juniper berries, which is perhaps why it is a drink historically associated with inducing early abortions.

The treatment of herbs and their association with careless malpractice is a historical one. John Actour was fined and imprisoned on several occasions throughout the 1600s. He kept repeat-offending and being punished, due to the fact that he was a surgeon and, as such, believed, unfoundedly, that this gave him licence to administer medicines. During his third charge, which was actually for murder, Actour failed to turn up to the hearing. Amazingly, the verdict ended up as deferred and then 'incomplete'.[62] Another repeat-offender was Francis Anthony, a medical physician practising in London throughout the early 1600s. Despite allegedly 'curing' in excess of twenty people, he had no licence to do so. Francis went to prison several times for his crimes: one woman lost all her teeth, for the death of a Captain Lee, for giving some sort of lethal pill to a person with epilepsy who was found dead three days later, killing a third person and leaving a fourth critically ill. In 1600, he was investigated and was 'in all parts of medicine … found inadequate in all'. He was denied permission to practise but continued despite going to prison, receiving fines and being publicly ostracized by his peers.[63]

Edward Aulding was both a medical practitioner and physician working in London between 1617 and 1641. Having been charged and cautioned in 1628, he went on to administer an enema containing saffron (bizarrely), a bezoar (a solid mass of indigestible material) and the root of serpentaria (Virginia snakeroot), to a servant of a Mr Alsope, called Gillman Scott. Scott died shortly afterwards and the autopsy revealed stones in the man's lungs. It looks like Edward Aulding panicked and accused Alsope of murdering his servant by kicking him to death. The autopsy ruled this out but Aulding failed to turn up to court, which meant the case never came to trial.[64]

It would seem that being absent from court often meant freedom to continue practising illegally. Sometimes leniency was granted, even during the 1600s which is not a period particularly known for its compassion. Susanna Gloriana was a French immigrant accused of murdering Mary Brett in 1602 after giving her a 'purge of syrup of hyssop and roses' followed by a herbal bath. Mrs Brett died six days later, although no information was provided regarding her illness. Gloriana confessed but the court fined her £20 and her case was referred to the French church in London. She was reprieved due to her state of poverty, being pregnant and having a newborn baby to take care of.[65]

Skilled silk weaver Matthew Desilar was not so lucky. In 1595, he confessed in court to prescribing a Mrs Noble 'a weak syrup of poppies, anise, cumin and cammomile' for a heart condition and treated a Mrs Willigis for a wasting disease using white dead nettles. It is unclear whether either died but Desilar was sent to prison.[66]

The media chronicles countless examples of malpractice by qualified doctors throughout history. Prior to the formation of the National Health Service, being treated for an illness and being admitted to hospital were subject to payment schemes which were complex and varied depending on the period. During the nineteenth century and into the twentieth, female almoners would assess the social background of the person being treated to determine an affordable fee. Hospitals were also institutions which many working people from poorer backgrounds feared. If you had money you paid for a private doctor; if you did not have money your options were limited to the local or recommended cheap quack. It is hardly surprising then that so many people turned to alternative and more affordable methods of treatment, even after the dawn of medical science.

Strewers and Sellers

Herb strewers were employed to distribute herbs and flowers in the royal apartments, or for other noble purposes including weddings, special events and so on. The primary reason for this was an attempt to mask the unpleasant aromas of the day. There are records stretching back to early medieval times, but by the regency period it was a profession in decline.

In 1901, Miss Beatrice Fellowes, daughter of Rear Admiral Butler Fellowes, became a victim of a new court ruling to abandon outdated offices such as armour-bearer and bow-bearer and so on. She had been selected as chief herb strewer by Edward VII for his impending coronation. This was based on Beatrice's hereditary responsibility, coming as she did from a long line of royal herb strewers. Her predecessor, another Miss Fellowes, had performed the task, along with six of her assistants, at the coronation of George IV when she cast rosemary and other sweet-smelling herbs across his path as he walked between Westminster Hall and the Abbey.[67] A lady called Alice Bell was a herb strewer for George I and her uniform must have been quite luxuriant, as records from the Lord Chamberlain's office describe the purchase of 'two yards of scarlet cloth for a livery for the year 1716'.[68] This scarlet outfit would have had the king's cypher embroidered on it.

Mary Dowle was herb strewer to King James II's first wife, during her coronation in 1685. As was tradition, she was assisted by six other young ladies, who wore hooded cloaks, holding one basket between two of them. They were dressed in full costume, with deep pointed bodices, open robes and exposed petticoats, with long ruffled gloves. Nine baskets of sweet-smelling herbs were said to have been strewn during the ceremony.[69]

Farmers' wives on country estates were responsible for cultivating the strewing herbs and a visit to England by Dr Levinus Lemmius in 1560, recounted in *Harrisons Description of England in Shakespeare's Youth*, was quoted saying:

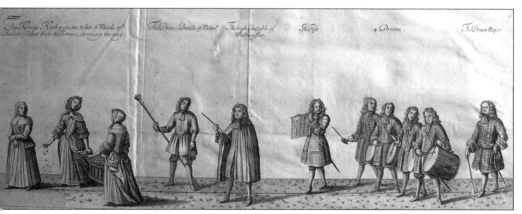

Herb strewing during the coronation procession of King James II and Queen Mary of Modena, c. 1685.

And beside this, the neate cleanliness, the exquisite finenesse, the pleasaunt and delightfull furniture in every poynt for household, wonderfully rejoiced me; their chambers and parlours strawed over with sweet herbes refreshed me.[70]

Adorning households with seasonal herbs has long been an English pastime. Samuel Pegge's *Curiala* describes aspects of the hospitality received at the court of King Stephen in the eleventh century, which he suggests would have been crowded with both nobility as well as tenants and those of inferior rank, who were regularly fed in rooms where the floors were 'strewed with flowers', a custom Pegge confirms was standard practice. The venerated twelfth-century Archbishop of Canterbury, Thomas à Becket, gave daily orders for his hall to be strewn with fresh hay or straw in the winter and with freshly gathered green leaves in the summer. This was partly to accommodate any visitors who had to sit on the floor.[71]

Writer Hugh Plat, who was also known for his culinary works in the sixteenth and early seventeenth centuries, advised:

for summer-time your chimney may be trimmed with a fine bank of mosse … or with orpin, or the white flower called everlasting. … And at either end one of your flower or Rosemary pots. … You may also hang in the roof and about the sides of the room small pompions or cowcumbers pricked full of barley, and these will be overgrowne with greene spires, so as the pompion or cowcumber will not appear. … You may also plant vines without the walls, which being let in at quarrels, may run about the sides of your windows, and all over the sealing of your rooms.[72.]

Herb Sellers

In the accounts of 1489/90 in Clerkenwell Priory the notice to quit rent amounting to 6s. 8d. from Nicholas Norton's tenancy was not received, leaving the tenement vacant and enabling local herb sellers to trade; this would have been an opportunistic venture for early herb street sellers, who were at this time also operating in nearby St. Pancras at a location simply called 'le Erbewywes' (the herb wives) [73] In 1631 'herb wives', along with oyster wives and tripe wives, were charged with the title of 'unruly people', during a time when hawkers, pedlars, street-sellers, itinerants – however you chose to define them – were denounced for their trades. Established traders and shopkeepers were threatened by the street-sellers who worked alongside them in direct competition and towards the end of the seventeenth century a new law was even introduced in which many were punished with fines or whippings. Costermongers continued to ply their wares, despite the penalties and thrived in Victorian London until the shopkeepers undercut them to such an extent that they were simply no longer able to continue trading.[74]

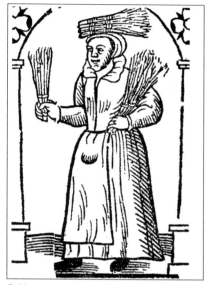

Selling rosemary and bays from Samuel Pepys's *Cries of London*.

The cries of London street-sellers are documented in the broadside ballads of the time, known as the *Roxburghe Ballads*. That of a herb seller in 1759 reads:

> Here's fine rosemary, sage, and thyme.
> Come, buy my ground ivy.
> Here's featherfew, gilliflowers and rue.
> Come, buy my knotted marjoram, ho!
> Come, buy my mint, my fine green mint.
> Here's fine lavender for your cloaths,
> Here's parseley and winter savory,
> And heartsease which all do choose.
> Here's balm and hyssop and cinquefoil,
> All fine herbs it is well known.
> Let none despise the merry, merry cries
> Of famous London Town.
>
> Here's penny royal and marygolds.
> Come, buy my nettle-tops.

Here's water-cresses and scurvy grass,
Come buy my sage of virtue, ho!
Come, buy my wormwood and mugworts.
Here's all fine herbs of every sort.

Here's southernwood that's very good.
Dandelion and houseleek.
Here's dragon's tongue and wood sorrel,
With bear's-foot and horehound.
Let none despise the merry, merry cries
Of famous London Town.[75]

In the 1670s, Gideon Harvey recommended purchasing herbs from the 'physical herb women' located in London's markets, where a handful of herbs would set you back half a penny (about 20p). This was on the proviso that you were unable to grow them in your own garden at home. For other more exotic spices he recommended a trip to the grocers.[76]

By the end of the 1700s, Covent Garden was known as 'the greatest market in England for herbs, fruit and flowers'. The herb shops and exclusive fruiterers were located in the south row, with the florists on the west side and roots and kitchen garden produce positioned on the north side of the market.[77] The North of England also had a significant network of itinerant herb sellers by this period. Manchester boasted sixteen organized market-based herb sellers in 1801, Leeds had eleven and Northampton seven, to name a few. The Parker family of Lancashire were renowned for their herb business, growing their own wares on an industrial scale for commercial trading. At least twenty-three herb growers, cultivating specialist herbs between 1790 and 1820, have also been identified in the north-west of England.[78]

Based on the census returns of 1841 and other documents, interestingly there are only two herbalists and one herb distiller listed in the whole of Scotland, with none whatsoever employed in either of these occupations in Ireland in 1847.[79]

There are quite a number of documented accounts of herb sellers being arrested for disorderly and drunken behaviour, using bad language and so on across the media during the Victorian era.

Like many other street vendors life would have been tough. Reformist and journalist of the day, Henry Mayhew, clarified that most London herb street-sellers of the Victorian era were Irish women, who traded from stalls during the autumn and winter months. One of these sellers was interviewed as part of Mayhew's documented observations, quoting:

Thrade isn't good, sir; it falls and it falls. I don't sell so many herrubs or so much ciliry [celery] as I did when mate [meat] was higher. Poor people thin, I've often been said it, used to buy bones and bile them for broth with ciliry and the beautiful herrubs. Now they buys a bit of mate and ates it without brothing. It's good one way and it's bad another. Only last Saturday night my husband – and a good husband he's to me, though he is a London man, for he knows how to make a bargain – he bought a bit of mutton afore the stroke of twelve, in Newgit-markit, at 2 ½ d. the pound. I don't know what parrut it was. I don't understand that, but he does, and tells me how to cook it. He has worruk at the docks, but not very regular. I think I sill most parrusley [parsley]. Whin frish herrings is chape, some biles them with parrusley and some fries them with ing-uns. No, sir; I don't make sixpence a day; not half a crown a week, I'm shure. Whin herrubs isn't in – and they're autumn and winter things, and so is ciliry-I sills anything; gooseberries and currints, or anything. If I'd had a family, I couldn't have had a shoe to my futt.[80]

This account provides a good deal of information relating to the decline in popularity of herb sales, in part due to the reduction in the price of meat. By the 1860s and '70s, the labouring classes in particular, no longer needed to flavour scraps and bones to make a decent broth when they could buy a proper cheap cut of meat. We are also given a stark reminder of how herbs were once seasonal, when today most herbs can be consumed all year round. The sale of herbs was becoming obsolete. This particular herb seller made somewhere in the region of between £1 and £1.50 a day in modern currency. Mayhew himself wrote that the once thriving street trade in agrimony, balsam, wormwood, tansy and so on to make medicinal teas, flavour puddings (tansy) or moth preventatives (wormwood) was no longer evident.

Mayhew interviewed a vendor of medicinal cough drops and other medical confectionery. This particular seller had a barrow stall in Holborn, selling dried horehound and coltsfoot and a variety of herb candies that were sold in stick form. His narrative is similar to the herb seller:

The cough drop and herb trade is nothing now to what it was long ago, it was as good as 3L. or 4L. a week to a person and was carried on by respectable men. I know nothing of any 'humbugs' in the respectable part of the trade. What's done by those who are ignorant and not respectable, is nothing to me. I don't know how many there were in the trade thirty or forty years ago; but I know that, ten or eleven years since, I supplied seven persons who sold cough drops, and such like, in the streets, and now I supply only myself and another. I sell only four or five months in the year – the cold months, in course; for, in the summer, people are not so subject to coughs and colds. I am the 'original' maker of my goods. I will cure any child of the whooping cough, and very speedily. I defy any medical man to dispute it, and I'll do it – 'no cure, no pay.' … Perhaps the wives of mechanics are among my best customers. They are the most numerous, but they buy only ha'porths and penn'orths. Very likely, they would think more of the remedy if they had to pay 13 ½ d. for it, instead of the 1 ½ d. The Government stamp makes many a stuff sell. Oh! I know nothing about quackery: you must inquire at the stamp-office if you want to know about them kind of medicines. They're the people that help to sell them. Respectable people will pay me 1s. or 2s. at a time; and those who buy once, buy again … I can dispel wind in two minutes. I sell bottles too for those cures (as well as the candy from herbs); I manufacture them myself. They're decoctions of herbs, and the way to prepare them is my secret. I sell them at 2d. to 1s. … I sell herbs too, but it's not a street ale: I supply them to orders from my connection. It's not a large trade. I sell horehound for tea … coltsfoot for smoking as herb tobacco (I gather the coltsfoot myself) … hyssop for wind, and Irish moss for consumption.[81]

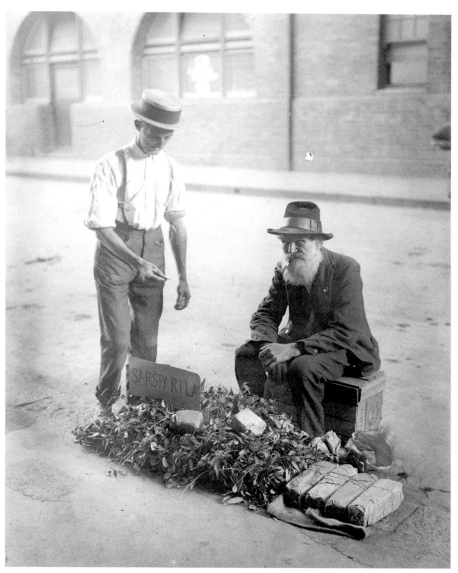

State Library of New South Wales, Sydney markets, by Rex Hazlewood, c. 1911–16.

By the start of the twentieth century the role of herb sellers and practitioners had become clearly defined, with practitioners having to serve a seven-year apprenticeship, before passing an exam.[82] It is evident from Mayhew's interviewee that government legislation was impacting on the livelihoods of the old street sellers, sifting out the 'humbugs' – people who tricked consumers into buying something that was not legitimate –

much earlier than this. The seller of medicinal wares suggests a previous salary for his trade of somewhere in the region of £150 which was a far cry from the 50-odd pence he was making for single street remedies, around 1860.

Hospitals, Gardens and Stores

Although forests were cleared for grazing and crops, differentiating what was a garden or simple farm land in Iron Age Britain is largely speculative. The earliest of structured gardens in England were forged by the Romans; large villa and palace gardens were a mix of landscaped greenery, formal designs, box hedges, statues and ornaments often with a small kitchen garden. Undoubtedly Anglo-Saxon communities would have carried on this tradition; with literary references of the time, including Bald's *Leechbook*, *Aelfric's Colloquy*, the writings of Bede and others providing a degree of knowledge relating to plants generally and their medicinal and culinary value.

During the Middle Ages, basic infirmaries were attached to ecclesiastical buildings, which were in turn attached to physic gardens, where a myriad of healing herbs were grown. As the centuries progressed, a similar practice grew out of the purpose-built urban hospitals. These

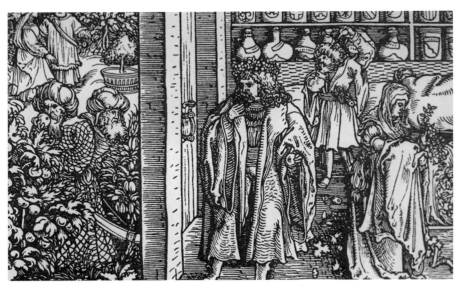

1915 reproduction print of a medieval herbalist's garden and storeroom.

would invariably have included some form of herb store, providing regular access to dried herbs with which to treat patients. Early versions of these 'open hospitals' fell under the remit of medical monks, most of which sprang up during the twelfth century, including:

Clerkenwell Hospital of Knights of St. John
Cirencester Hospital of Knights of St. John
Westminster St. James's Hospital for Lepers
St. Bartholomew's Hospital
St. Alban's St. Mary's Infirmary
St. Alban's Road, St. Julian Leper Hospital.
Winchester St. Cross Hospital
Northampton, Hospital of Knights of St. John
Ripon, St. Mary's Hospital
St. Katherine's Hospital, London
Hospital of St. John, Bath
Sherburn Leper Hospital, Durham
St. Opportune Hospital, the monks of St. Katherine, Durham
St. Thomas's Hospital, London Bridge.[83]

One such store, which incredibly still exists, is the Herb Garret, now part of a museum which includes the Old Operating Theatre of St. Thomas's Hospital in London, the oldest surviving surgical theatre in Europe. The oak-beamed attic directly above St. Thomas' Church was built in 1703 and it was used to store medicinal herbs to be administered to patients in the hospital. One of the herbs you would undoubtedly have seen in large quantities in the garret at that time was wormwood. This was a herb so named for its supposed abilities to cure one of the deadliest ailments in London – parasitic worms. Chamomile, a well-known sedative, was also commonly used by surgeons as an antiseptic during some procedures.[84]

London's Chelsea Physic Garden was originally designed as a training ground for apothecaries who needed to study and identify herbs for treatments. It was founded by the London Society of Apothecaries in the 1600s. Originating in 1617, the Worshipful Society of Apothecaries remains one of the largest of livery companies still in existence today. Basically, apothecaries were early pharmacists, born out of the medieval Grocers' Company, whose primary purpose was to prevent the adulteration

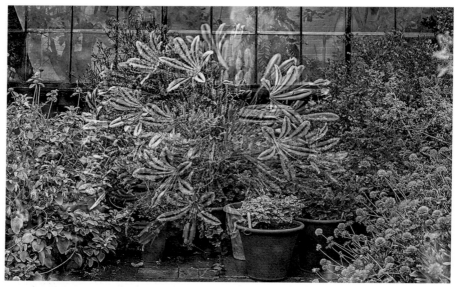

Chelsea Physic Garden greenhouse.

of drugs and spices. Resenting the restrictions outlined by the Grocers' Company, Huguenot rebel Gideon de Laune led a breakaway group of apothecaries to form a new society with a remit to train apprentices and ensure medicines were regulated.[85]

In 1673, the society rented several acres of land in Chelsea, which they enclosed with a brick wall, while additional funds were raised to grow herbs. By 1678, 150 pounds of mint were provided to be distilled as an oil, along with sage, pennyroyal, sweet marjoram and rue. A series of gardeners were recruited from the dishonest and eventually dismissed Spencer Piggott, to Richard Pratt who liaised with fellow gardeners at the oldest botanic garden in Britain: University of Oxford Botanic Garden, with a legacy that extends to 1621. Oxford's first director, Jacob Bobart the elder, published a list containing around 1,400 plants from the garden, in 1648, titled, *Catologus plantarum Horti medici Oxoniensis* (*Catalogue of the Plants in the Oxford Medicinal Garden*).

Several species from that same book are still grown in the garden today.[86.] Other notable historic English physick gardens of this period include Petersfield Physic Garden, founded around 1681, and Edinburgh in 1670.

By 1680, John Watts was managing the gardens at Chelsea and it is due to his input that the garden began to develop a more international approach to cultivating new foreign species. This same year the first greenhouse was built, swiftly followed by a heated house which may well have preceded earlier known ones built in Holland around this time. Watts's ground-breaking work was followed by Samuel Doody and James Petiver, who produced vast lists of plants alongside detailed descriptions.

Unable to find the funds to buy the freehold for the land, Sir Hans Sloane stepped in as a member of the committee and by 1722 he had become the new landlord, using monies secured from the wealth he had accumulated in Jamaica. Conditions of Sloane's generous agreement with the Society of Apothecaries was to maintain scientific progress and to ensure the preservation

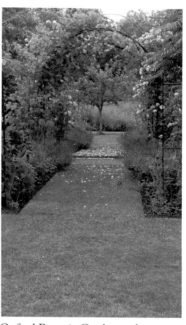

Oxford Botanic Garden and Arboretum. (*Emma Kay*)

of different species. Sloane also introduced gardener Philip Miller to the society, a man who would ultimately raise the profile of the physick garden forever. He introduced rare plants, liaised with botanists globally and developed the cotton trade in America by sending the long-strand cotton seeds he cultivated across the Atlantic to the new colony of Georgia.[87]

The second oldest physick garden in the country, Edinburgh, has a delightful link to the historical narrative of rhubarb cultivation in Britain. Professor John Hope was keeper of a section of the Royal Botanic Garden in Edinburgh in 1760. His colleague, Dr James Mounsey, trained at Edinburgh University and set up his own private practice in Moscow, eventually becoming a royal physician to Catherine the Great and Tsar Peter III. Following the suspicious death of the Tsar (perhaps plotted by Catherine and her lover), Mounsey was put in an awkward position and managed to get Catherine to retire him on the grounds of ill health. He smuggled several pounds of rhubarb seeds from St. Petersburg Botanical Gardens, founded in 1714, back to Edinburgh in 1762. This was an act that would have been punishable by death, as rhubarb cultivation was

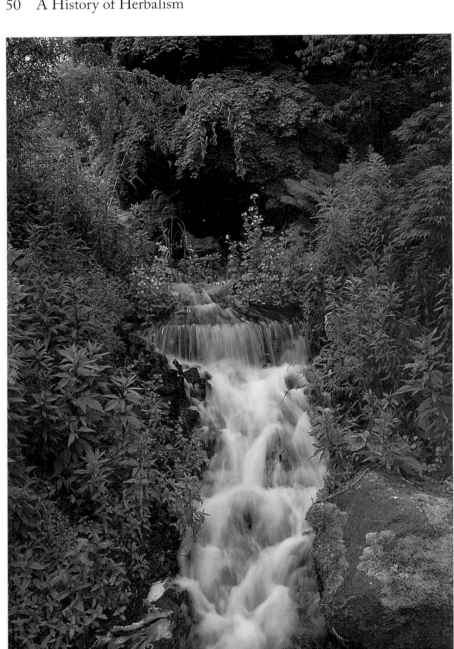

Waterfall, Royal Botanical Garden, Edinburgh.

highly prized in Russia, providing a substantial income in exports. Mounsey moved to Dumfriesshire in 1763 where he would have had to reside in hiding for the rest of his life and was awarded a gold medal by the Royal Society of Arts in London in 1770 for the role he played in introducing Russian rhubarb into Britain. His colleague, Sir Alexander Dick, acquired some of Mounsey's rhubarb seeds and cultivated them at Preston Field House, now a luxury hotel in Edinburgh, where incidentally, you can still find the 'Rhubarb' restaurant in its grounds. Mounsey's other trusted colleague, Dr John Hope, cultivated the seeds, both at the Royal Botanic Garden in Edinburgh and at Kew Gardens.[88]

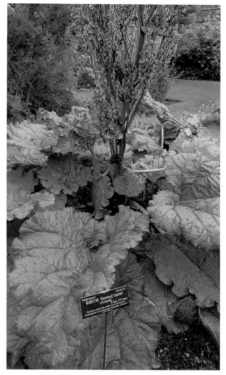

Rhubarb at Oxford Botanic Garden and Arboretum. (*Emma Kay*)

Herb Illustrators

If you have ever drooled at the exquisitely beautiful sketches of herbs and plants in early botanical publications, then this section of the chapter aims to provide a little context behind some of those talented artists.

Woollen draper turned botanical artist, Sydney Parkinson was born in Edinburgh in 1745 and moved to London to become more proficient in the art of drawing. It was here that he trained with botanist Joseph Banks, mostly drawing plants at Kew Gardens, before joining Captain James Cook, on Banks's recommendation, on his extraordinary circumnavigation of the globe. Whilst sailing on HMS *Endeavour* from 1768 to 1771, through South America, Tahiti, New Zealand and Australia, Parkinson produced at least 1,300 drawings and paintings.[89] As well as his wonderful sketches, Parkinson left behind his journals which reflect some of the adventures the crew encountered on their *Endeavour* voyages, like this extract written just after leaving Papua New Guinea:

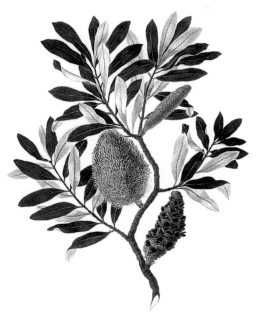

Sydney Parkinson *Banksia integrifolia* watercolour from Banks's *Florilegium.*

A party of our people went, in the pinnace, to examine the country while we stood off and on. They soon returned with an account that a great number of the natives threatened them on the beach, who had pieces of bamboo, or canes, in their hands, out of which they puffed some smoke, and then threw some darts at them about a fathom long, made of reeds and pointed of Etoa wood, which were barbed, but very blunt. Our people fired upon them, but they did not appear to be intimidated; our men, therefore, thought proper to embark. They observed that these people were not negroes, as had been reported, but are much like the natives of New Holland, having shock hair, and being entirely naked. They also saw plenty of cocoa-nuts growing on the trees, as well as lying in heaps on the ground; and plantains, bread-fruit, and Peea [sic].

And of the herbs in the South Sea Islands:

This sort of purslain grows very common in the low islands, where the inhabitants bake and eat it, and account it very good food.

Parkinson's journal cuts short towards the middle of January 1771, when another voice presents itself to announce:

On the 16th of January, we took our departure from the island, and a few days after, the disorder with which several of our company had been attacked, and died at Batavia and Cooper's Island, began to rage among us with great violence, and in a few days, carried off Mr. Charles Green, the astronomer, Mr. Sydney Parkinson, Mr. David Spoving, clerk to Mr. Banks, and many of the common men.

Sydney Parkinson died of dysentery in January 1771 on board the *Endeavour*. He was just 26 years old.[90]

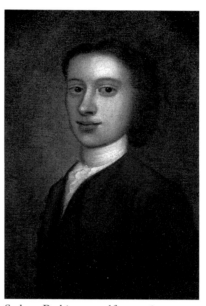

Sydney Parkinson, self-portrait.

Ann Lee, was tutored by Sydney Parkinson during his time in London. Sydney also bequeathed all his painting and drawing paraphernalia to Ann in his will – a wish which was sadly intercepted by Parkinson's employer, Joseph Banks, who managed to acquire all of Parkinson's possessions. Some of these were redistributed by John Fothergill following a public attack against Banks in the media, by Sydney's brother Stanfield.

Ann's father, James Lee, was a Scottish gardener and apprentice to Chelsea Physick Garden's, Phillip Miller. Undoubtedly inspired and influenced by her father, Ann was commissioned by English physician and plant collector John Fothergill to create a series of flower paintings on vellum. These are now housed at the Royal Botanic Garden, Kew.[91]

Marianne North was a Victorian plant hunter and prolific botanical painter. We know something more of her life due to the fact that she kept diaries and wrote *Recollections of a Happy Life: Being the Autobiography of Marianne North*, which was published by her sister after her death.

In 1867, Marianne noted that the family had abandoned London for most of the season, preferring instead to devote themselves to their garden in Hastings where her father constructed three glasshouses: one for orchids, one for 'temperate plants' and 'one quite cool for vines and cuttings'.

Marianne talks about frequently visiting both Chiswick Gardens and Kew Gardens to paint the flora and flora. Following a brief period

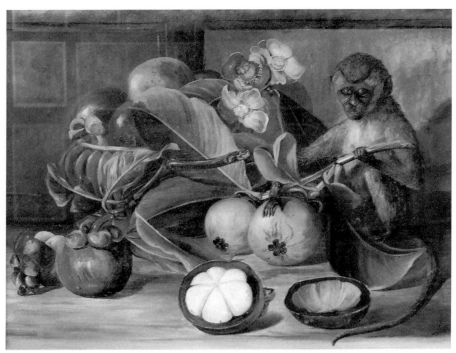

Flowers and fruit of the mangosteen, and Singapore monkey, by Marianne North.

travelling together with her father across Europe and Syria before he became too ill to continue, dying in 1869, Marianne had made the decision to travel overseas to document, collect and record tropical plants. She visited Jamaica alone in 1871/2, a brave and unusual undertaking for her status, age and gender back then. She was overwhelmed by the experience declaring: 'I was in a state of ecstasy, and hardly knew what to paint first.'

But it would be just the first of many endeavours. Marianne travelled to Jamaica, Brazil, Tenerife, California, Japan, Singapore, Borneo, Java, Ceylon, India, Australia, South Africa, the Seychelles and Chile, embracing all her cultural experiences with gusto and passion. She was finally forced to retire to Gloucestershire in ill health, before dying in 1890. Marianne has several plant species named in her honour.

She opened a gallery to exhibit her work at Kew Gardens in 1882, which was restored in 2008. Marianne was an extraordinary woman and one of the last botanical illustrators to capture rare and exotic plants before the onset of popular photography.[92]

In stark contrast, Ebenezer Sibly was an eighteenth-century physician, astrologer and writer of the occult. He was also the engraver of Culpeper's first illustrated copy of *The English Physician*, published in 1789.

Sibly was a white supremacist who believed that humans had not inhabited Africa until much later in history, believing categorically that the continent's first communities were white. He argued that native Africans had become black as a consequence of the hot climate. Sibly was also a Master Mason. In his book *A Key to Physic* he talks at length about the properties of various herbs, linking their appearance to the appropriate ailment. For example:

> Herbs which resemble the lungs, promote respiration, and strengthen the lungs, as hounds-tongue, lung-wort, sage, camphorey, wall-wort etc. … herbs which resemble the nose, as water-mint, etc. So plants that bear resemblance with the womb, conduce much to strengthen and comfort the same, to purge the uterus, and promote fecundity, as the round birth-wort, briony, ladies-seal, heart-wort, Satyrium and mandrakes, which hath round and hollow roots.

Perhaps akin to his opinions on race, Sibly also believed in 'English herbs for an English constitution'.[93]

One woman who made the very most of understanding the wildlife of Africa was Northamptonshire-born Katharine Saunders (née Wheelwright) who relocated to South Africa with her husband in 1854 at the age of thirty.

She spent her early life in Tansor with her six siblings, mother and father, Canon Charles Apthorp. Katherine was painting watercolours by the age of 6 and as an older teenager she studied drawing on the

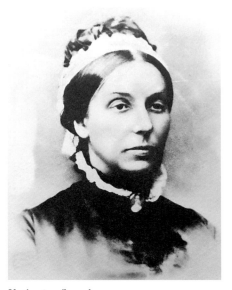

Katharine Saunders.

continent, becoming proficient in numerous languages on her travels. She met her husband, James Saunders, while in Brussels and they were married in 1851. Finding work difficult to obtain in England, the family, including their young daughter, moved to South Africa, where James's employers, the Natal Company, had invested in sugar plantations.

With Scotsman and curator of the Durban Botanic Garden, Mark Johnston McKen, as her mentor and tutor, Katherine began painting, identifying and recording as many unknown species as she could, while liaising with Kew Gardens and the keeper of the herbarium at Trinity College, Dublin. She became well known as a botanist in her own right in eastern South Africa. In later life Katherine travelled extensively across South Africa's rugged terrain, always sketching and collecting samples along the way. She was a tough, determined avant-garde illustrator and unsurprisingly spent time with kindred spirit Marianne North, who stayed with the Saunders during her three-week stay in Natal in 1882. Of the 426 specimens Katherine sent to Kew between 1881 and 1889, at least sixteen were named after her including *Schrebera saundersiae*. [94]

The most contemporary botanical illustrator of this chapter is Arthur Harry Church who died in 1937. An academic and lecturer at Oxford University, Arthur was born in Plymouth, Devon, and his drawings are still considered to be some of the finest compositions ever to be drafted in the UK. Hundreds of his original watercolours are housed in the permanent collections of the Natural History Museum. He was made a fellow of the Royal Society in 1921.[95] In 1915, Arthur lost both his daughter and his wife within a couple of months of each other, leading to a breakdown, one perhaps he would never really fully recover from. His photographic studies of plants represent an early pioneering area of work in this field and he was one of the few botanical artists to traverse the arts of hand-drawn and photographic botanical images in the early twentieth century.[96]

Chapter 2

Magic and Medicine

'Nature ... She will hang the night with stars so that I may walk abroad in the darkness without stumbling, and send the wind over my footprints so that none may track me to my hurt: she will cleanse me in great waters, and with bitter herbs make me whole.'[1]

For centuries magic and medicine were intwined before the application of herbs for secular treatments became a more formal method of dispensing medicine. While the previous chapter outlines the chronology of British herbalists and medical practitioners, this part of the book will provide a guide to the individual herbs themselves, listing their uses and properties from enchantments to pharmaceutic applications.

Britain has historically integrated the use of herbs into all manner of practices, cultural and religious, influenced by a wealth of different sources, from prehistoric remedies to medieval 'physick' gardens and astrological herbology. Rituals and incantations once accompanied the dissemination of herbal remedies, with the healing power of herbs being just as likely to be used to fend off evil powers as to protect or bewitch. The first section of this chapter will investigate the magical elements of herbs, the plants and roots that were once associated with magic for spiritual and physical wellness, and those used as talismans or for more sinister purposes.

While a herbal tea might have offered you a peep into the future, some ancient magical systems relied on the waning of the moon or the position of the stars to ensure a herbal charm was successful. Certain herbs were also more effective if they were enchanted first, which could be achieved as they were being picked, or by visualizing the goal in mind when being handled. Other herbs worked better when tied in bags or sachets and some as 'poppets' or dolls were crafted in human form, a practice most associated with voodoo. Mandrakes are a good example of this.

An infusion was simply a case of soaking herbs in water before being drunk directly or rubbed into the recipient's possessions, whereas bathing in herbs or herb oils enabled the complete absorption of the remedy or spell to dissolve into the skin. Other herbs were best burnt and used as an incense or made into ointments.[2]

Another important charm used in herb magic is the amulet, from the Latin *amuletum*, an object that drives away unwanted forces, while protecting the recipient. Roman author and philosopher Pliny the Elder wrote avidly about the use and composition of amulets in his magnum opus, *Natural History*. He affirmed that almost anything could be crafted into an amulet, which needed to be attached to the neck or limbs. Pliny nominated the combination of cyclamen root and basilisk blood (a species of lizard) as the ultimate protection against evil spirits and bats.[3]

The remaining half of this chapter provides an A–Z of medicines, treatments and cures associated with specific herbs. Typically headaches and joint pains were once treated with herbs that had a sweet countenance like rose, lavender and sage, while wormwood, mint and balm soothed a myriad of stomach conditions; liquorice and comfrey were used for the lungs and vinegar and myrrh for cleaning and sanitizing wounds.[4]

Ancient remedies ranged from the conventional to the bizarre. The Massachusetts Historical Society once owned a significant collection of old medical recipes which included a remedy for smallpox, in which toads were required, but only toads collected in the month of March. They were then boiled and pounded down in a mortar with other plant life.[5] Adders and vipers were also thought to contain medicinal powers and were regularly used in early medicine. As outlined in the introduction, the properties of herbs and their relationship to the physical world have been carved out of thousands of years of ancient philosophical musings and our closest interpretations of these can be gained from the translations and re-imaginings of the medieval era. Walahfrid Strabo, who died around AD 849, became abbot of Reichenau, in south-west Germany; he composed a poem titled, *The Little Garden* which represented a sort of guide to monastic medicine. It is very detailed and based on Walahfrid's own knowledge and wide understanding of the medicinal application of herbs. The following excerpts from Walahfrid's work are taken from Raef Payne's 1966 translation of *Liber de cultura hortorum* and provide a nice introduction into the world of individual herbs and the powers they were once so highly bestowed:

Horehound

  Horehound comes next, and what shall I say of this.
Powerful worker? A precious herb though biting
And sharp on the tongue where it tastes so unlike.
Its scent: for whereas the scent is sweet, the taste.
Is not sweet at all. Yet taken in a draught,
For all its nastiness it assuages pain
In the chest, and most when drunk still warm from the fire
And ladled out quickly to close the meal.
If ever
A vicious stepmother mixes in your drink
Subtle poisons, or makes a treacherous dish
Of lethal aconite [wolfsbane or monkshood] for you, don't waste a
  moment –
Take a dose of wholesome horehound; that
Will counteract the danger you suspect.

Fennel

  Let us not forget to honour fennel. It grows
On a strong stem and spreads its branches wide.
Its taste is sweet enough, sweet too its smell;
They say it is good for eyes whose sight is clouded,
That its seed, taken with milk from a pregnant goat,
Eases a swollen stomach and quickly loosens
Sluggish bowels. What is more, your rasping cough
Will go if you take fennel-root mixed with wine …

Chervil

  Come, hoy Muse, thou who in sacred song
Canst stablish monuments of mighty wars
And mighty deeds – come, scorn not to touch with me
The humble riches that my garden yields.
Now chervil, though it splits and divides itself
In flimsy branches and gives but a paltry seed
In its thick clusters of ears, yet flourishing
All the year through gives largesse to the poor
And comfort.

A draught of this, so easy to take,
Will counter and check internal bleeding. Again,
When mixed with pennyroyal and poppy leaves
It makes a poultice which will prove effective
For a stomach that's upset and racked with pain.

Pennyroyal

   The humble scale of my song will not allow me
To embrace in fleeting verse the many virtues
Of pennyroyal. They say that Eastern doctors
Will pay as much for it as we pay here
For a load of Indian pepper. Since such a people,
Rich as they are, blessed with gold and ebony,
Who give to an eager world a wealth of marvels-
Since they will buy at such a price, so greedily,
Our pennyroyal, who can doubt its power
To allay a host of troubles?
Oh, how wise,
How good is God! Let us praise him as we ought.
From no land he withholds his bounty; what is rare
Beneath this sky, under another lies
In such abundance as the cheapest trash
We have among us here: some things we scorn
Rich kingdoms pay great prices for. And so
One land helps another; so the whole world,
Through all its parts, makes one family.
Believe me, my friend, if you cook some pennyroyal
And use it as a potion or a poultice, it will cure
A heavy stomach – that you can take for truth.
Some things are only hearsay, but custom and usage
Allow us to blend them in with lofty truth – like this:
When the sun is blazing down on you in the open
To prevent the heat from harming your head, put a sprig
Of pennyroyal behind your ear …
Ah me!
If my impatient Muse were not now forcing me
To take in sail and make at last for harbour,
Many another flower could I gather for you.

Betony

> In the mountains and woods, in the meadows and depths of the valleys,
> Almost everywhere, far and wide, grows the precious abundance
> Of betony. Yet I have found it too in my garden, and there
> It learns a softer way of life in the tended soil.
> So great is the honour this genus has won for its name
> That if my Muse wished to add to it she would find herself
> Defeated at last, overwhelmed; and soon she would see
> She could add nothing more to the value it has already.
> Perhaps you pick it to use it green, perhaps
> To dry and store away for the sluggish winter.
> Do you like to drink it from cloudy goblets? Or do you
> Prefer to enjoy what it gives after long and careful
> Refining? Whatever your fancy, the wonderful powers
> Which this herb has will supply all your needs.
> Indeed, some men I know rate it so highly
> That, hoping to find protection from every harm
> That assaults the inner body, day after day
> They drink a dose of this harsh but soothing tonic.
> Again, if your head is cut and the wound turns septic,
> Crush some sacred betony, make of it dressings
> And apply them frequently: you will be amazed
> How quickly its powerful influence closes the wound.
> And here in handsome rows you can see my agrimony.
> It clothes all the fields with its profusion; it grows
> Wild in the woodland shade. Much honour it has and many
> Virtues – among them this: if it's crushed and drunk
> The draught will check the most violent stomach-ache.
> And if an enemy blade happens to wound us
> We are accustomed to try its aid, pounding
> The shoots and putting them on the open place.
> If we remember to add to the dressing some sharp
> Vinegar, our full strength will soon be restored …[6]

Similarly, the *Lacnunga*, which roughly translates as 'remedies', is a collection of medicinal recipes and charms compiled mostly in Old

English and Latin. Written around the same time as Walahfrid Strabo's guide to monastic medicine and bearing great similarities is the Anglo-Saxon poem called the *Nine Herbs Prayer* (or *Charm*). It contains a mixture of pagan and Christian elements citing the most powerful herbs of that time: mugwort, plantain, bitter cress, betony, chamomile, nettle, crab apple, chervil and fennel, along with instructions on how to prepare them for use. Translated it reads:

Artemisia Vulgaris [mugwort]
Remember thou, Mugwort, what thou declared
What thou advised at the proclamation of the gods [*Regen* 'council
    of the gods' and *meld* 'proclamation']
Una [First] thou were named, the eldest of *worts* [herbs]
Thou hast might against three and against thirty,
thou hast might against venom and against that which flies.
thou hast might against the loathsome that yond the land fareth.

Plantago Major [plantain]
And thou, *Waybread* [plantain], mother of worts
open to the east, mighty within;
over thee carts creaked, over thee queens [women] rode,
over thee brides cried out, over thee bulls snorted.
All of them thou withstood and dashed against;
so may thou withstand venom and that which flies
and the loathsome that yond the land fareth.

Cardamina Hirsuta [hairy bittercress]
Stune [watercress] is named this wort, she on stone waxes;
stands she against venom, *stuneth* [dasheth] she against pain.
"Stiff" she is named, withstandeth she venom,
wreaked [driveth out] she the wrathful, *warpeth* [casteth] out venom.

Stachys Annua [betony]
This is the wort that with *wyrm* [serpent] fought,
she that prevails against venom, she that prevails against that which
    flies,
she prevails against the loathsome that yond the land fareth.

Put thou now to flight, *Adder-loather* [betony], the lesser [and] the
  more
the more [and] the lesser, until he, of both, is cured.

Matricaria Discoidea [chamomile]

Remember thou, *Mayweed* [chamomile], what thou declared,
What thou earned at Alder-fjord;
that never for that which flies life would be *sold* [given, lost]
since for him mayweed, as *meat* [food], was readied.

Urtica Dioica [nettle]

This is the wort that is named *Weregulu* [nettle];
this sent a seal over the sea's ridge
the undoing of venom, to others a cure.

Malus Domestica [crab apple]

These nine have *main* [power] against nine venoms.
Wyrm came sneaking. It slit a man
Then took up *Wóden nine glory-tines* [tines of Wuldor],
slew with them the adder that she into nine flew.
There earned Apple and venom
that she never would *bend-way* [slither] into house.
Anthriscus Sylvestris [chervril], Foeniculum Vulgare [fennel]
Chervil and Fennel, most mighty two,
those worts were shaped by the witty Drighten,
holy in the heavens, where he hung;
set and sent [them] into seven worlds
for the wretched and the wealthy for all a cure.
Stands she against pain, *stuneth* [dasheth] she against venom,
that prevails against three and against thirty,
against the fiend's hand and against *far-braiding* [shape-shifting?],
against *maskering* [bewitching] by evil wights.
Now prevail these nine worts [herbs] against the nine wonder-
  flying-ones,
against nine venoms, and against nine which fly,
against the red venom, against the foul smelling venom,
against the white venom, against the blue-grey venom,

against the yellow venom, against the green venom,
against the *wan* [dark] venom, against the *woad* [blue] venom,
against the brown venom, against the crimson venom,
against the wyrm-blister, against the water-blister,
against the thorn-blister, against the thistle-blister,
against the *ice-blister* [frostbite], against the venom blister,
if any venom comes flying from the east,
or any other from the north, any [from the south] come
or any other from the west over the tribes of men.
I alone *wot* [know] of a river running
There the nine adders near it *beholdeth* [keep watch];
May all weeds now from worts spring,
Seas to slip away, all salt water,
When I, this venom from thee blow.

The charm to cure infection:

Mugwort, *Waybread* [plantain] that is open to the east, *lambcress* [stune], *adder-loather* [betony], mayweed, *nettle* [Weregulu], apple, chervil and fennel, and old soap: work the worts to dust, mix with the soap and with the apple's gore. Work up a slop of water and of ashes, take the fennel, *well it up* [boil it] in the slop and bathe it with an egg-mixture, when he dons the salve, either ere or after. Sing that *galdor* [incantation] o'er each of those worts thrice ere you work them and on the apple also; and sing it into the man's mouth and in both ears and on the wound likewise galdor, ere he dons the salve.[7]

Herbs and Magic A–Z

Aconite/Aconitum is second only to mandrake in its powers. With its beautiful helmet-shaped purple flowers, aconite is more commonly referred to as wolfsbane or monkshood; it is, together with mandrake, thought to represent the link between the human and plant world. Wolfsbane is also associated with banishment, the banishment of undesired visitors, including both humans and spirits.[8] As its alias wolfbane suggests, it is synonymous with the plant's legendary abilities to repel fantastical beasts such as werewolves. Aconite can be highly toxic, but, thanks to

Dr Storck's experiments on himself during the 1760s, he confirmed that it could be safely consumed in the right quantities. Incidentally, Storck also advocated the positive benefits of another poisonous plant, hemlock, to cancer patients.[9] The French physician Paul Étienne François Gustave Curie, who was also the grandfather of pioneering scientist Pierre Curie, was an advocate of homeopathic medicine, writing widely on the subject. He claimed that for easing the symptoms of pleurisy, characterized by the inflammation of the lungs, there was 'no remedy superior to Aconite'.[10]

Adder's root/tongue or **arum** is also highly toxic, but has been used to relieve eczema and ulcers if prepared by an expert. Its appearance is startling and often referred to as resembling male or female genitalia. Robert Johnson was a celebrated Elizabethan musician and composer, who worked in the Royal Court and for William Shakespeare. His name has been linked to a score titled *The Masque of Queens*, which was undoubtedly used in original performances to accompany the three witches in Shakespeare's *Macbeth*. Shakespeare included numerous descriptive names of plants in his work, as herbalism was so integral to society in the sixteenth century. It is possible to interpret the infamous words in Act IV, Scene I of *Macbeth*:

> Eye of newt and toe of frog, Wool of bat and tongue of dog, adder's fork [adder's tongue] and blind-worm's sting, Lizard's leg, and howlet's wing [henbane].

Robert Johnson's composition may also have accompanied the poem and masque performance of the same name by Ben Jonson. Written in 1609 for Queen Anne, it depicts the story of twelve witches who reveal a stream of vile crimes, while dancing and cavorting, before being interrupted by twelve more virtuous queens. Jonson wrote:

> The Scrich-owls Eggs, and the Feathers black,
> The Blood of the Frog, and the Bone in his back, I have been getting;
>   and made of his Skin A purset, to keep Sir Cranion in.
> A Nd I ha'been plucking [plants among]
> Hemlock, Henbane, Adders-tongue,
> Night-shade, Moon-wort, Libbards-bane;
> And twise, by the Dogs, was like to be tane.[11]

There are a number of nineteenth-century literary references to arum being used as a substitute for orchid bulbs in the manufacture of saloop, a popular alternative to tea and coffee in England during the eighteenth and nineteenth centuries. This drink has a legacy which is both Arabic and Roman in origin, as an intended aphrodisiac. (See Chapter 3 for a saloop recipe.)

Agnus Castus is the name given to the tree Vitis Agnus Castus, which was regarded as a symbol of chastity, largely because of confusion between the Greek term for this tree and for the term 'chaste'. The seed had a small place in early modern medicine, but it has only been noted once among apothecary inventories. It is a flowering Mediterranean tree and is widely regarded as a successful herbal treatment for hormonal imbalances. Its magical attributes are linked to chastity and fertility. According to Nigel Pennick, medieval monks ate the berries of the tree in order to supress their libidos, hence its nickname 'Monk's pepper'. [12] It was familiar to ancient Greek physicians and written about by philosophers, conversely as both an aphrodisiac and a means of supressing sexual desires.

Agrimony or **church steeples** grows widely in Europe, North America and Japan with flowers resembling mini yellow spinning tops which blossom from June to September. It is primarily a diuretic, but it was once used as a protective herb to fend off witches and bad spirits. It played an active role in breaking hexes, as well as protecting people from having hexes put on them and shielding troubled sleepers from bad dreams and unwanted night time visitors. Perhaps this is one of the reasons why it has become associated with the promotion of sleep. [13]

Alfalfa is classified as both a legume and a herb and has always been linked to prosperity. This is perhaps because farmers have been able to successfully cultivate it in abundance for centuries and it can greatly enhance soil fertility. It was sometimes kept in jars in the home to ward off poverty and hunger.[14]

Alyssum: there are many species of this pretty flowering plant that grows in a range of colours and is also known as madwort. Pedanius Dioscorides endorsed alyssum as a cluster of flowers that could be made into an effective amulet, writing as he did of this plant: 'Pounded together in meat and given, it is thought to cure madness in a dog' and 'Hanged on them with a purple cloth, it drives away sores on cattle'.[15]

Angelica: as well as its healing qualities, the root of angelica was singled out by John Gerard, a man who scrutinized and rejected the occult, as something that could be carried around to protect against witchcraft and enchantments in the sixteenth century.[16] Some people protected their properties with angelica, by sprinkling it into every corner; it has also been used by Native American tribes as a gambling talisman.[17]

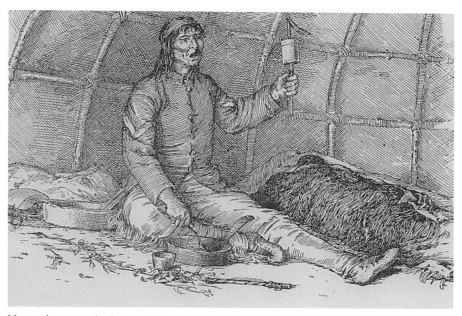

Native American herbalist, 1880.

Basil, most notably **Indian basil,** or **tulasi,** is regarded by Hindu cultures as a herb which protects against all misfortunes, guarding against disease and injury. It is also believed to safeguard children from ill health.[18] Basil is apparently still administered for stomach cramps in China, but is far more of a culinary herb these days. According to Cornelius Agrippa's early sixteenth-century compilation, *Occult Philosophy*, garden basil rubbed together between two stones had the power to produce scorpions, because it was ruled by celestial Scorpio.[19] Apparently, when the Romans cultivated basil, no doubt sowing the seeds far and wide throughout their imperial onslaught, they cursed and abused the seeds. This was based on an ancient assumption that the more you damned the plant, the more it yielded.[20]

Bay leaf: in England a withered bay leaf was once considered an omen of death, with William Shakespeare writing in *Richard II*:

> Tis thought the King is dead; we will not stay.
> The Bay-trees in our country are all withered.[21]

Bay leaves come from several bay trees, including the bay laurel, which is why it is often confused with laurel trees. The word laureate, to describe someone who is honoured highly, is a derivative of laurel. Hence the trend for ancient Greek and Roman leaders to wear wreaths of laurel to demonstrate their authority and why Shakespeare also associated its decay with the demise of King Richard II. Bay leaves have been more commonly used as a culinary herb since at least the early 1600s.

Belladonna, the **deadly nightshade,** means beautiful lady and, as such, it is often, in the world of magic, associated with improving one's

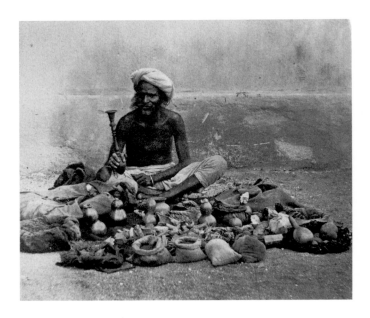

Indian medicine
seller, 1862.

appearance. It is extremely toxic and is harvested for the purposes of poisoning. The leaves of belladonna were once applied to the skin to ease ulcers and tumours.[22] Giambattista della Porta claimed that one drachm (⅛ of a fluid ounce) of belladonna root could 'make men mad without any hurt, so that it is a most pleasant spectacle to behold'. Whether this was of equal entertainment for the man as well as the spectators is not clear. But caution was given by stressing the need to not increase the dose, which could stimulate 'alienation of minde for three days'. Quadruple the dose and you would not live to experience another hallucination.[23]

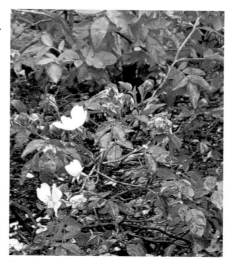

Deadly nightshade. (*Emma Kay*)

Betony root traditionally provided an excellent cure for headaches. This herb, which at one time grew in abundance in meadows and shady areas, was considered a shield against 'monstrous nocturnal visitors and Frightful visions and dreams'. Betony was thought to have the power to make snakes 'lash themselves to death' if a circle of the herb was placed around them.[24]

Black hellebore: Culpeper listed black hellebore as a herb which was astrologically guided by Saturn. All herbs under this particular ancient Greek category were associated with strengthening properties. Culpeper suggested it should be administered with 'greater safety after being purified, than when raw', adding that 'Country people use it for such beasts as are troubled with the cough … by boring a hole through the ear and putting a piece of the root therein'. It was also commonly given to people with mental health disorders in medieval times, as Saturn was of a melancholic nature.[25]

Bryony: as this plant was formerly believed to be governed by Uranus, it became synonymous with warding off lightning. The first Roman emperor, Caesar Augustus, wore a wreath of bryony leaves to protect himself from lightning during military campaigns.[26] So, it clearly wasn't just laurel/bay leaves which we typically associate with being worn around the heads of Roman victors.

Castor oil plant: when hung up in the house the castor oil plant was once thought to redirect hail storms away from a property, as well as preventing ships entering storms when the plant was placed on board. It was, however, essential that you were completely clean when you picked it, or its charms would prove ineffective.[27] Ricin is the highly toxic poison produced in the seeds.

Chicory: the sixteenth-century German occultist Henry Cornelius Agrippa believed that the star formation of Ursa Minor, or the 'Little Bear', ruled over chicory, the leaves and flowers of which are said to grow towards the north, in the direction of the seven-starred constellation's position in the northern sky.[28] If gathered and cut using a gold knife, in total silence at noon or midnight during midsummer, chicory was also gifted with the power to open locked doors or boxes.[29]

Chives: in Central Europe bunches of dried chives were at one time hung around the house, suspended from the ceilings or doors to ward off evil spirits. Apparently in some regions of Holland in the nineteenth century, farmers fed their cows on chives to flavour the milk.[30] While in China, Buddhist monks excluded chives from their diet, along with other vegetables from the Allium family such as onions and garlic, as they are traditionally thought to stimulate the passions.[31]

Cinquefoil: the unique mystical qualities of the herbaceous flowering plant, cinquefoil (five-leafed), became the insignia for some of the medieval crusaders, who carried shields bearing a single cinquefoil. Only those considered capable of gaining full control of the five senses – hearing, sight, smell, taste, touch – were allowed to wear this emblem. It represented the highest of orders.[32]

Coriander or **Chinese parsley** or **cilantro**. A little trick of sewing coriander seeds into clean linen clothes, which when firmly pressed onto the inner left thigh of either the man or woman in a relationship trying to conceive, was once believed to stimulate their fertility.[33]

Chamomile: in parts of Germany, formerly Prussia, chamomile flowers were gathered on the eve of St. John's Day and made into wreaths which were placed in houses to protect against ravaging storms.[34] Chamomile was dedicated to the mother of the Virgin Mary, St. Anne. The word itself is a derivative of a Greek word meaning 'earth apple'. Traditionally, it was grown in alleys and walkways and on the banks of rivers, as it was understood that the more chamomile plants were pressed and trodden down, the more abundantly they would grow.[35]

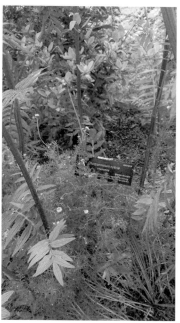

Chamomile at Oxford Botanic Garden and Arboretum.
(*Emma Kay*)

Cress: a fragment from *Nineveh*, a seventh-century Assyrian medical compendium, alludes to the symptoms of witchcraft, including anything from continuously coughing up white phlegm, to vomiting and pains in the chest and shoulders. One of the suggested cures includes mixing cress with other plants such as juniper and soapwort, crushing and sifting them together, before adding the mix to beer and cedar oil and smearing it on the enchanted person.[36] Watercress, or lamb's cress is also one of the plants featured in the ancient *Nine Herbs Prayer*.

Feltwort or **mullein** was valued highly as a remedy for all aspects of respiratory problems. It also had a reputation as a herb which kept wild beasts of all descriptions away, if you kept a twig of it on your person. By all accounts, feltwort was so powerful it could ward off any form of evil.[37]

Fennel was regarded as a symbol of false flattery, exemplified in Robert Greene's *Quip for an Upstart Courtier* (1592): 'Fennell I meane for flatterers.'[38] In the Middle Ages the seeds of fennel were used as an appetite suppressant for fasting pilgrims. As a consequence, it became a symbol of something that appears to sustain, but actually is completely ineffectual. Snakes were thought to be able to cure their own sore eyes by eating fennel as well as using it to shed their skins. A medieval spell containing fennel was understood to protect people against elves, unwanted nocturnal visitors and eerily, women known to have had carnal relations with Satan. It involved the following method:

> One takes the ewe hop plant, wormwood, bishopwort, lupin, ashthroat, henbane, harewort, viper's burgloss, heatherberry plants, cropleek, garlic, grains of hedgerife and fennel. These herbs are put in a vessel and placed beneath the altar where none masses are sung over them. They are then boiled in butter and mutton fat; much holy salt is added; the salve is strained through a cloth; and what remains of the worts is thrown into running water. The patient's forehead and eyes are to be smeared with this ointment and he is further to be censed with incense and signed often with the sign of the cross.[39]

Foxglove was traditionally applied as protection against fairies.[40] In Wales the leaves of the foxglove were used to make a black dye which would be painted in crossed lines on the floor, near the entrance of the house, to prevent any evil from entering the property.[41]

Garlic: moly or **sorcerer's garlic** has ancient associations with magic. In Homer's *Odyssey*, it is the herb given to Odysseus to protect him from wizardry. As Hermes passes the herb to the hero of this epic poem, Odysseus exclaims:

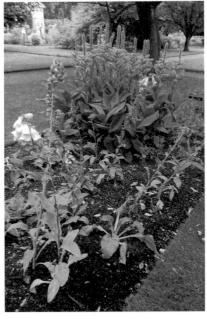

Foxglove at Oxford Botanic Garden and Arboretum. (*Emma Kay*)

Its root is black and its flower white as milk
And the gods call it moly. Dangerous for a mortal man
To pluck from the soil but not for deathless gods.
All lies within their power.[42]

John Gerard also touches on its abilities to drive away diseases and mentions moly as a plant known at the time for conjuring witches and bestowing enchantments, both activities which he condemns as 'foolish' and 'vain'.[43] According to Richard Folkard writing in the nineteenth century, if you dreamt about eating garlic you would be destined to discover hidden secrets, while dreaming about garlic being in the house meant the dreamer would be blessed with good luck.[44]

Hemlock is alleged to have been the herb used to poison Socrates. It was also used in a series of murders in the United States in the 1930s, to kill over 100 men poisoned by their wives, who then cashed in their insurance policies. The syndicate behind these deaths provided the women with the poison and then collected their fee following the insurance payout.[45] Every part of hemlock contains a volatile poison called conia, a drop of which is sufficient to kill a small animal. The poison finds its way to the spinal cord, producing paralysis and convulsions. The contents of the witches' brew in Shakespeare's time-honoured and dark tragedy *Macbeth* contains among other ingredients once considered nefarious, 'Root of hemlock digg'd i' the dark'.

Henbane is a poisonous plant which has a legacy of being used in magic to encourage love. If a man desired to fall in love, he needed to gather henbane early in the morning, while standing on one foot and then wearing the plant in order to attract love.[46] Henbane, along with pennyroyal, chervil, vervain, poppies, mandrakes, hemlock, and dittany were all generically used by witches when making spells, according to Rosalind Northcote.[47]

Hellebore is a member of the buttercup family, of which there are around twenty species, the most recognized being black hellebore and white hellebore. Both are highly poisonous. During medieval times black hellebore was used in conjunction with other ingredients to abort babies. Hellebore was a plant applied regularly as a means of balancing bodily humours (hot, cold, dry, wet). As with many other poisons, when consumed, hellebore will induce vomiting and diarrhoea, which is probably why it was considered to make such an excellent purgative.[48] More ominously in medieval witchcraft, hellebore was present during exorcism rituals and used in conjunction with spells designed to seek revenge.[49]

Hempseed: John Houghton claimed that 'Hempseed is good to make hens lay often in the depths of winter'.[50] In parts of Cornwall and Derbyshire on Valentine's eve and midsummer's eve respectively there was a practice involving young girls, who on the stroke of midnight, would visit a churchyard, run around scattering hemp seed while repeating the following chant:

> I sow Hemp-seed: Hemp-seed
> I sow
> He that loves me the best
> Come after me and mow.

The purpose of this invocation was designed to secure a future husband.[51]

Henna: the Greeks once used henna as a shampoo, which they created by pounding its leaves together with the juice of soapwort.[52] Traditionally in India the flowers of henna are used to repel moths and there is a superstitious notion that when the flowers are in bloom, both snakes and men converge around women.[53]

Herb bennet or **colewort** or **avens** was viewed as a very positive herb. Known originally as St. Benedict's herb, it was named after the eponymous saint, whose cup was poisoned with wine, but shattered into pieces before it could be drunk. As a consequence, the plant became associated with antidotes.[54] Confusingly colewort is also a brassica, a different species of plant altogether, which was eaten in abundance during the medieval period as a cabbage, consumed independently or in pottages.

Horehound: according to the ninth-century monk Walafrid Strabo, horehound was an excellent antidote to evil spells and concoctions. He wrote: 'If some evil stepmothers mix up poisonous substances and slip them into your drink, or deceptively load lethal wolfsbane into your food, then quickly down a draught of the antidote horehound and you will soon be rid of the anticipated dangers.'[55]

Juniper berries were previously burnt at funerals in Britain to ward off evil spirits. Ancient pagan rituals included the application of incense acquired from the smoke of its burning green branches.[56]

Lavender: believe it or not, lavender is actually classified as a herb and not a flower. The eleventh-century abbess, visionary and botanist, Hildegard of Bingen wrote about lavender in her compilation on the scientific and medicinal properties of nature, *Physica*. She stressed its inedibility, but owing to its strong aroma, she believed it had the potential to kill lice on people, in addition to fending off 'many evil things'.[57] The Grocer's Company of London, which once encompassed all of the city's apothecaries and sellers of herbal medicines cultivated a garden near their hall in Cheap ward around 1413 which was stocked with roses, thyme and lavender to provide London's wealthy entrepreneurs with a place to escape the stressful commercial aspects of the city.

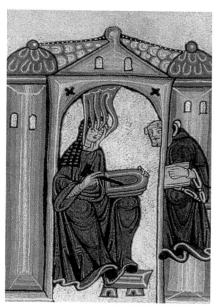
Hildegard von Bingen.

Larkspur: if someone was unlucky enough to have been suffering with a fever for four days or more, the answer apparently was larkspur and peppercorns. The peppercorns had to be added as an odd number. For example, grind thirty-one peppercorns with larkspur on day 1, on day 2 use seventeen peppercorns and thirteen on the third day and so on. The fever apparently should break shortly after this ritual.[58]

Lupin: together with bishopwort, henbane and crop leek, according to the eleventh-century *Leechbook*, is a herb once used to rid people of demonic possession. Pounded together and mixed with ale and holy water the concoction had to be drunk out of a church bell to be effective. Lupin was also used in combination with other herbs in spells designed to resist temptation.[59]

Mandrake: Henry Maundrell. the respected academic and clergyman who famously travelled from Syria to Jerusalem, documenting his accounts along the way, observed that in some Arab nations right up until the seventeenth century, it remained customary for women who wanted to conceive to lay mandrakes under their beds.[60] Mandrake was also once widely used as a narcotic. In Shakespeare's great historical love story, *Antony and Cleopatra*, the Egyptian queen requests, 'Give me to drink mandragora … That I might sleep out this great gap of time my Antony is away.'

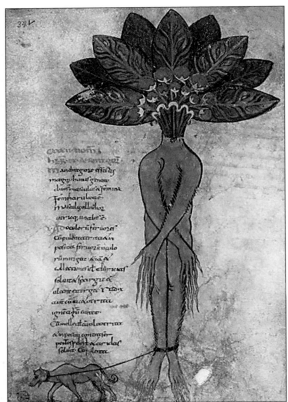

Kassel mandragora (mandrake) from the ninth-century version of *pseudo apuleius herbarius.jpg*.

During the 1880s, Benjamin Ward Richardson made detailed studies of the mandrake, mixing the root with alcohol and water. His experiments on small animals left them sedated and after consuming it himself he recorded numbness of the tongue, a dry mouth, blurred vision and an oversensitivity to sound. He praised the mandrake for its anaesthetic properties and believed it could help relieve tetanus.[61]

As the mandrake visually resembles the lower part of the human body, it was common for street vendors in seventeenth-century London to sell 'mannikins', which were marketed as sentient plants, to complement spells and potions. This was a practice that John Parkinson, Charles I's herbalist, believed to be misleading to the public, calling for an end to the charlatan street hawkers in his book, *A Garden of All Sorts of Pleasant Flowers*.[62] Parkinson did, however, recognize the anaesthetic properties of the root. In the Middle Ages throughout Europe people, particularly women caught in possession of a mandrake could easily be accused of witchcraft, with some hanged or burnt at the stake, just for having it in their possession.[63] The shrieking mandrakes depicted in the Harry Potter films, are based on the sound that they make being removed from the ground, which has widely been exaggerated over the centuries, to include screams and groans, adding to the mandrake's reputation as a sensate object. In Germany it is called *Zauberwurzel* (sorcerer's root) and young girls from rural communities wore bits of mandrake around their necks as love charms.[64]

Pseudo-Apuleius's fourth-century *Herbarius*, which was republished across the centuries, is the oldest known written herbarium. A version of this manuscript from the ninth century depicts the mandrake in its humanized form, a popular early medieval image.

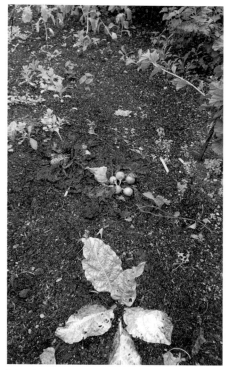

Mandrake roots at Oxford Botanic Garden and Arboretum. (*Emma Kay*)

Melissa aka **lemon balm**: in seventeenth-century Germany, alleged witch Barbara Schleicher was found in possession of a sack of roots and herbs including melissa, hellebore and juniper, three herbs that were associated with black magic and poison. Being in her possession, this was used as strong evidence to convict her of witchcraft. Although lemon balm can bring on drowsiness and affect pregnancy, it must at one time have been linked to much greater malevolent activities in Renaissance Germany.[65] Roman philosopher Pliny, advocated the use of lemon balm for healing wounds, as he believed it stopped the flow of blood. In some eastern cultures it was believed to influence the power of love.[66]

Mermaid weed or **proserpinaca**: according to Bald's *Leechbook* the best remedy for sore eyes was to make your way over to a patch of wetland harbouring mermaid weed, just before sunrise or sunset (assuming you could see it in such an uncomfortable state). Then while scratching the undergrowth around the herb, using a ring of gold, you simply requested the soreness to abate. It was then a case of waiting for three more days (after which having sore eyes for that long, presumably you might be worried), before returning to pick the weed and string it around your neck. Voilà! No more sore eyes.[67]

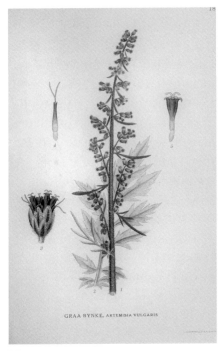

Motherwort or *Leonurus cardiaca*– is part of the mint family and Culpeper declared 'it makes women joyful mothers of children'. According to him one spoonful in a glass of wine alleviated what we would probably now refer to as Postnatal depression.[68]

Mugwort was also known as 'oblivion', particularly in France where its association with memory loss was understood to convince travellers to lose their way.[69] Placed in the shoe, mugwort was also believed to help weary travellers when accompanied

Mugwort.

by the words, 'I will take thee artemisia, lest I be weary on the way' before making the sign of the cross.[70] One can only surmise that if travellers possessing mugwort were always getting lost, additional quantities of this herb would serve to ease their tired feet in the process.

Myrtle is a protective herb, once considered to be the luckiest plant to reposit in your house. It has also long been recognized as a symbol of love, dedicated to Aphrodite.[71] *Hoodoo – Conjuration – Witchcraft – Rootwork* is a slightly eccentric and eye-opening series of lengthy volumes which document the oral histories of diverse former and practising witches. In one of these volumes an interview revealed mixing snakeroot, oak bark, and myrtle root together in alcohol, making a colourless and odourless poison – one that could kill.[72]

Nettles: *Petit Albert* is a grimoire attributed to Albertus Magnus of the 1700s which became a huge publishing success due to its affiliation with devil worship. It is filled with spells and rituals, one of which includes a technique to determine whether a poorly patient will live or die:

> Take a nettle and place it in the patient's urine, incontinent after the patient has made it, and so that it shall not be contaminated at all, and leaves the nettle in said urine for the space of twenty-four-hours; and after if the nettle is found dry, it is a sign of death; and if it is found green, it is a sign of life.[73]

One berry or **Paris herb** or **true love herb** was once a highly prized medicinal herb, believed to expel poisons and toxins from the body, including the plague. One berry was labelled a plant associated with witchcraft on account of its potency. It grows abundantly in woods and copses in Britain and has a powerful root system.[74]

Parsley: the German physician and scholar Henry Cornelius Agrippa, writing in the early 1300s, recounted how parsley, linseed, flea-bane seed and violets mixed together into a fume, had the potential to enable whoever was mixing the concoction to foresee and prophesize the future.[75]

Chap. 527.   *English Herbs.*   789

XIV. *The Fricasie.* The first Kind, or both the sorts, being Fried with Eggs, as you Fry *Clary Leaves*, and so eaten, it is said to be a singular Medicine to cure the Weakness of the Back.

XV. *The Cataplasm.* Being made of either of the Green Herbs, and applyed to places affected with the Gout, it cools, eases the Pain, stops the afflux of Humors to the Part; and in some reasonable time cures the Patient.

es and Fibres *spreads it self under the upper Crust of the Ground, something like a Couch-Grass Root, but not so white, and not much lesser than the Root of the White Wild Anemony, or Wind-Flower, and almost of as dark a color, being much like thereto in its creeping. This Root shoots forth Staks with*

One Berry: or, Herb True Love.

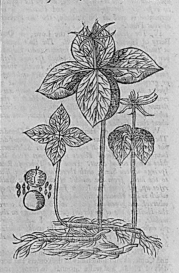

CHAP. DXXVII.

Of ONE BERRY;

OR,

HERB TRUE LOVE.

I. **THE *Names.*** It knows no *Greek* Name: But the *Latines* call it *Herba Paris*, and so it is generally called by all *Herbarists*; and in *English*, One Berry, *Herb True Love*, and *Herb Paris*. Some have thought it to be a kind of *Aconitum*, but were deceived, and therefore *Fuchsius* called it *Aconitum Pardalianches*, and *Cordus* seems to be of the same Opinion, and therefore calls it *Aconitum Pardalianches monococon*, they accounting it to be dangerous and deadly: but *Matthiolus* contradicts all this, for that it has been found by Experience, not to be hurtful but Salutiferous, for which reason *Tabernæmontanus* called it *Aconitum Salutiferum*, which yet I think to be an improper Name also, for that it is no Species of the *Aconites*. Some have thought it to be a kind of *Aster*, or *Starwort*, and therefore *Tragus* called it *Aster sed non Atticus*, but it is no Species of the *Starworts:* he also called it *Uva Lupina*, and *Uva Canina*. Others have thought it to be a Kind of *Solanum* or *Night-shade*, but it is no more a Species of that Plant than it is of the two former; but upon this supposition *Pena* and *Lobel*, in their *Adversaria* call it *Solanum Tetraphyllon* (from the form of the Leaves and Berry:) and *Bauhinus*, as leaning to the same Opinion, *Solanum quadrifolium Bacciferum*; both of which so call it very improperly: and I think the first Name *Herba Paris*, is the fittest we can bestow upon it.

II. *The Kinds.* There are three Species of this Plant very well known, *viz.* 1. *Herba Paris vulgaris*, *Herba Paris Tetraphyllos*; Our Common Herb True Love or One Berry. 2. *Herba Paris Floridensis*, *Herba Paris Floridiana, vel Brasiliana*, *Herba Paris Triphyllos Brasiliana, Solanum Tryphyllium Brasilianum Bauhini*, Herb True Love, or One Berry of *Florida*, or of *Brasil*. 3. *Herba Paris Canadensis radice rotunda, Herba Paris Floridensis radice tuberosa: solanum Triphylium Canadense Cortusi*, Herb True Love of *Canada*.

The Descriptions.

III. *The first*, or Our Common Herb True Love, or One Berry. *Has a Root which is long and tender, small and creeping under the Earth, dispersing it self hither and thither; its Taste is Styptick or Astringent, and very unpleasant, and by its Branch-*

Leaves, *some of which bear no Berries, and some do, every Stalk being smooth, without Joints, and of a blackish green color, rising to about six Inches high, if it bears its Berry; but seldom so high, if it bears none. This Stalk bears at the Top four Leaves, set directly one against another, in manner of a Cross, or a Cross-Knot, commonly called a True Loves Knot: which are each of them a-part, something like to a Night-shade Leave, but a little broader; and in some places, twice as broad as in others, for they oftentimes vary much. and tho' the stinted number of the Leaves is generally four: yet sometimes there are but three, and sometimes five, and sometimes six, which are sometimes smaller, and sometimes larger, and that by a quarter or half part, and sometimes they are (as is before said) twice as large. This Plant has been seen sometime to alter or degenerate, and that the four Leaves have not only been twice as large, as the ordinary, but they have also been dented in, both on the edges, and at the points, which have been parted, or forked, and have born larger Berries, than commonly this Plant is used to bear: all which are of a fresh green color, not dented about the edges. In the middle of these four Leaves, there rises up a small slender Stalk, about an Inch high, bearing at the top thereof, one Flower, spread open like a Star; consisting of four small and narrow long pointed Leaves, of a yellowish green color; and four other lying between them, lesser than they. In the middle whereof*

Woodcut of one berry or true love, taken from *Botanologia, the English Herbal*, 1710.

If for some reason you ever wanted to dissuade someone from staying in a house, the following charm which derives from 1930s New Orleans, using parsley, could provide you with a solution:

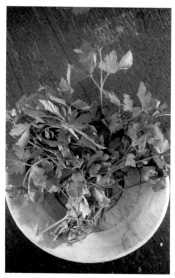

Parsley. (*Emma Kay*)

> Go out an' get yo' a bunch of green parsley, take yo' some chamber lye [urine that it is caught in a chamber pot] and get yo' a box of concentrated lye [caustic soda]. Yo' take dat parsley an' yo' put it on a fire, heat it until yo' kin pound it up. Yo' pound dat parsley up, yo' mix it up wit dat chamber lye, yo' mixes dat [concentrated] lye up with it, yo' puts it in a bottle, see. Yo' stops dat bottle up good an yo' turns dat bottle upside down, an' hides it in some place dere, conceal it where nobody will find it. I'll guarantee yo' nobody will ever line in dat house.[6]

Ragwort is a herb that can be poisonous to certain animals. Writing in 1669, Giambattista della Porta affirmed the important role this wild weed once played in terms of fertility, both the giving and taking away of virility and reproduction.[77] John Gerard also called this plant St. James, after its Latin name Herba S. Jacobi and classified it as both land and sea ragwort, with the sea variety being particularly abundant on the Isle of Sheppey. Gerard considered ragwort to be a dry and cleansing herb, on account of its bitterness. [8]

Rue: a documented folklore practice, which I cannot find a specific location for, involved young women making wreaths composed of rue, willow and cranesbill (a type of geranium). They then walked backwards to a tree, throwing the wreath over their heads until it caught on one of the branches and held fast. Every failed attempt to fix the wreath meant they would remain single for another year.[79] According to Culpeper, rue has an ancient association with chastity and the prevention of lewd thoughts.[80]

In Shakespeare's *Hamlet*, Ophelia, the prince's intended wife who loses her sanity towards the end of the play, distributes a selection of flowers and plants during a scene where she appears to be in a world of her own. She chooses a particular plant suitable to each character, but Shakespeare does not elaborate on the specifics of this:

There's rosemary, that's for remembrance.
Pray you, love, remember.
And there is pansies, that's for thoughts …
There's fennel for you, and columbines.
There's rue for you, and here's some for me.
We may call it 'herb of grace' o' Sundays.
– Oh, you must wear your rue with a difference.
There's a daisy. I would give you some violets,
But they withered all when my father died.

Some critics and later medieval interpretations suggest the rue was for Queen Gertrude, Hamlet's mother, a woman whose overt sensuality extends to insinuations of incest and adultery.[81]

Peony: William Langham, who was a medieval 'practitioner in phisicke', advocated using peony in the following way: 'The roote and seedes hanged about the necke of children, is good against the falling sickenesse, and the haunting of the Fairies and Goblins.'[82] A combination of dictionary and encyclopaedia scribed in Latin; the thirteenth-century book *Catholicon* was one of the first non-religious oversized volumes to be published. One entry refers to the Greek mythological *Lamia*, which was a creature with a human face and the body of a beast, a sort of female centaur. *Lamia* snuck into houses and tormented children. Many

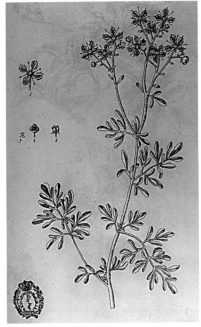

Sketch of rue from Elizabeth Blackwell's *A Curious Herbal.*

of the ancient leeches provide charms and nostrums to shield children from these types of 'elvys', just as Langham suggests.

Pennyroyal: according to Anglo-Saxon lore, if a woman miscarried it was believed a child could be revived by consuming three shoots of this herb, which required grinding down, before being mixed with aged wine.[83] This ancient member of the mint family is also well known in Greece for its abilities to help stimulate the menstrual cycle, linking it again to the course of pregnancy.[84]

Periwinkle had the potential to ward off demonic possession. It needed to be picked while chanting the following incantation, 'I pray thee vinca pervinca, thee that art to be had for thy many useful qualities, that thou come to me glad, blossoming with thy mainfulnessess; that thou outfit me so; that I be shielded and ever prosperous and undamaged by poisons and by wrath.' Like many herbs yielding special powers it was imperative that you were clean when you picked it, which had to be when the moon was nine nights old, then eleven nights, again at thirteen nights, thirty nights and lastly when the moon was again just one night old.[85]

Spiderwort, sometimes called misery, is an herbaceous perennial. An old fourteenth-century French manuscript yields a spell designed to treat a horse's hoof which has become damaged by a blacksmith's nail. According to the spell, by combining spiderwort and white bread and then feeding this to the horse two or three times a day, the horse will eventually recover from its wounds.[86]

St. John's wort: this ancient herb was once specifically cultivated as protection against tempests, thunder and evil spirits in Britain.[87]

Tansy: in Sussex people thought that by adding the leaves of tansy to the bottom of their shoes, it was possible to prevent fevers.[88] More frequently tansy was used in cooking (you can find a recipe in the following chapter).

Thyme: Lesley Gordon asserted that thyme was a herb which strongly identified with the afterlife. As such medieval women embroidered it

onto the clothing of knights to wear before a
tournament, as a symbol of bravery and to aid
courage.[89]

Tarragon is also known as the dragon plant, a
derivative of its French name *estragon*, thought
to counteract bites of venomous creatures. It is a
warm and fiery herb, which was once considered,
like thyme, to embody confidence and courage.
Tarragon was known to attract love and provide
protection.[90]

Verbena, also known as **ashthroat**, traditionally
warned off demons but could be used as part of
a rite which brought good luck and prosperity.
The following was recorded in the 1930s:

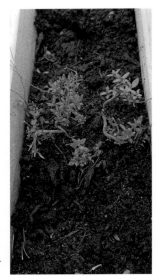

Thyme. (*Emma Kay*)

> Go to de drug sto' an' git essence of verbena an' fast luck, an' git a
> glass of watah an' put a silvah dime in it. An' git chew some – whut
> de name dat stuff yo' call it? … perfume dat's lucky, an' burn dat wit
> chure tapers fo' luck.[91]

Vervain: old English lore declared that if you wore this herb about
yourself, then dogs would never bark at you. Vervain was highly esteemed
by the Romans and was frequently offered as a pledge of peace or to
denounce war. [92]

Wormwood: in the previous chapter you would have read about
wormwood's abilities to treat parasitic worms. It was also once commonly
used in brewing and is best known perhaps by its other name of absinthe.
Common wormwood was supposed to counteract witchcraft and
necromancy. If a garland of it was thrown into the fire on midsummer
eve, accompanied by a sacred verse, it could protect a household from all
supernatural agencies throughout the year. [93] Henry Daniel wrote that
if wormwood was placed in the middle of a circle and a spider was then
placed next to it, the spider would most likely die. This suggests that
wormwood may also have been considered an early insecticide.[94]

Yarrow: according to Folkard, writing in 1884, yarrow was integral to several old charms, one of which centred around the South West of England, where young women seeking love would pick yarrow from the grave of a young man. It is a very ancient plant steeped in myth and legend. After picking the yarrow the girl would then be expected to say the following incantation:

> Yarrow, sweet yarrow, the first that I have found,
> In the name of Jesus Christ I pluck it from the ground;
> As Jesus loved sweet Mary, and took her for his dear,
> So in a dream this night, I hope my true love will appear.

The girl then slept with the yarrow under her pillow and in her dreams her husband would appear to her. [95] Apparently, yarrow was once found growing in abundance in churchyards, gaining it a reputation for driving the devil away.

Medicinal Herbs A–Z

Newcomb's Midland Counties' Almanac of 1866 provides a precise summary of instructions relating to the methods for preparing herbs for medicinal use. These include the following recommendations:

Juices
Which we are informed should be extracted by bruising herbs or roots in a stone mortar with a wooden pestle. The juice must then be set on a fire, skimmed to remove the scum and stirred continuously. The addition of oil to the juice once cold will help preserve the mixture.

Syrups
Herbs or roots should be bruised and boiled in water at the ratio of a handful of herbs to one pint of water. Reduce the mixture on the stove to half the quantity, cool and strain. Add half a pound of sugar to half a pint of the mixture; boil until a syrup is made. The syrup should be stored in a glass or stone bottle, with a cork or bladder seal and will last at least a year.

Ointments

Mix two handfuls of bruised herbs, flowers or roots with a pound with hog's lard and beat in a stone mortar. Place in a stone jar, cover with paper and set in a warm place until the fat melts. Boil gently and strain. Add another two handfuls of bruised herbs, leave to stand again and boil. Repeat until you have a good strong ointment. To every pound of ointment two ounces of turpentine and two ounces of wax should be added.

Poultices

Chop herbs or roots and boil in water until you get a jelly-like consistency. Add barley meal or oatmeal and some oil or suet. When ready to use, apply to a cloth and treat the area affected.

Decoctions

Are prepared in the same way as syrups. If wine is added they will last longer.[96]

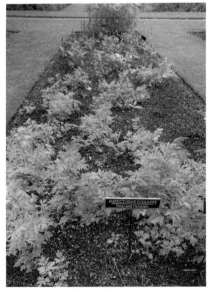

'Herbs for Viral and Parasitic Diseases', Oxford Botanic Garden and Arboretum. (*Emma Kay*)

Herbs have been used to treat ailments of all kinds since man's recognition of their natural healing properties thousands of years ago. Early texts and the musings of herbologists and botanists were based on the writings of Roman and Greek philosophers and scholars. But many of their individual medicinal identities have altered over the centuries. Writing in the seventeenth century, Nicholas Culpeper's pharmaceutical observations on burdock as an analgesic, for instance, that also eased excessive gas, differs greatly from its known modern-day antibiotic abilities to relieve skin diseases and soothe arthritis. He also classed bedstraw as an aphrodisiac when it is now used as a diuretic to help pass kidney stones.

Some interpretations of medical herbology have remained consistent. Recognized today as effective in alleviating gout, Culpeper once praised the herb pennyroyal while stressing its proficiency at relieving insect and snake bites. This is not dissimilar to its contemporary role as an insect repellent. Nonetheless, different botanists, herbalists and early physicians often contradicted each other with regard to the medicinal attributes of herbs and plants.

As a consequence, the inventory of medicinal herbs in the following section attempts to include a broad overview of the generic historical characteristics of herbs and their relationship to healing, within the framework of several centuries of observation from numerous gleanings.

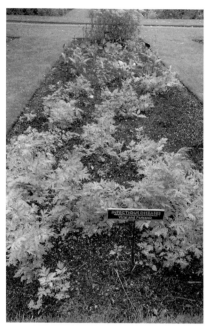

'Herbs for Infectious Diseases', Oxford Botanic Garden and Arboretum. (*Emma Kay*)

Aconite: the poison from aconite has many ancient uses, perhaps the most well known one being its long-standing relationship with whaling. Hunters have extracted the poison from the plant and rubbed it onto arrows and spears for centuries. Aconite, wolfsbane or monkshead, to name a few of its aliases, is a beautiful blue-flowering plant and one with a sinister past. Being both a neurotoxin and a cardiotoxin, death from aconite is an unpleasant one involving cardiac arrest and the paralysis of the body's entire respiratory system.[97] Nonetheless, its medicinal properties are also extraordinary. Early evidence from China's Western Han dynasty, as early as the second century BC in fact,

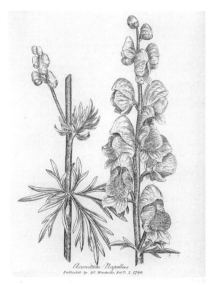

Aconitum, wolfsbane or monkshood, taken from Medical Botany Containing Systematic and General Descriptions with Plates from the BHL.

reveals medical formulas – over four hundred – have been excavated, revealing that aconite was the second most used drug, surpassed only by cinnamon. Aconite was applied externally and directly to wounds, skin disorders such as scabies and on abscesses. As time went on aconite was used to a greater extent internally to remedy the symptoms of colds, it was also mixed with other herbs and spices, such as liquorice and ginger to reduce its toxicity.[98]

Agnus castus: the berries of agnus castus are a small round fruit the size of a peppercorn, often a greenish brown or olive colour and are very bitter to the taste. According to John Hill, writing in 1751, the berries were a good remedy for 'hysterics' – the broad medieval term for women experiencing anything from anxiety, insomnia, bloating, reduced or heightened sex drive, irritability and any other symptoms we might today associate with premenstrual conditions, postnatal depression or menopause. For men, ingesting the berries could make them either sexually aroused or chaste, depending on the man.[99]

Agrimony: the seed drunk with wine was said to benefit the liver, in addition to its abilities to ease adder bites. Distilling its leaves in water relieved coughs, jaundice, fevers and cholick amongst other ailments.[100] The name agrimony derives from the ancient Greek word *Argemone*, 'cataract of the eye', as it was thought to heal cataracts and other visual complications. The Anglo-Saxons named it Garclive, while later medieval texts christened it Egrimoyne. It is still considered good for the liver today as well as aiding indigestion; it was frequently made into a tea, particularly in France, or used as a throat gargle.

Angelica has been cultivated in England since at least the mid-sixteenth century, becoming a highly prized addition to many gardens by the seventeenth century, as both a medicinal and culinary plant. Many published recipes of this time focus on candying or preserving it in syrup, or as a substitute for sugar. John Pechey, writing in his 1694 *Compleat Herbal of Physical Plants*, declared it a herb that had the ability to purge the body of poisons, recommending it as a cure for the plague. He also advised readers to eat the candied root or stalk of angelica every morning to prevent getting infections, to clear the lungs and alleviate bad breath.[101]

Balm, also known as **melissa** or **lemon balm** (the scent of lemons disappears when the plant is dried), yields an essential oil containing stearopten, which has a sort of resinous quality that can help speed up the healing process of some wounds. Pliny advocated the use of balm to treat headaches and nervous disorders, while Culpeper comments on its abilities to assist with stomach disorders. The 1822 edition of *The London Dispensatory* notes that while balm was once esteemed for its ability to aid 'nervous affections', it was at the time of writing, best known for reducing fevers when made into a tea.[102]

Basil was once dried and used in snuff, then taken to relieve headaches as well as being made into tea to encourage menstruation. Sweet basil was sometimes present during funerals, particularly in Iran and Keats's narrative poem *Isabella, or the Pot of Basil*, based on a fourteenth-century story, the eponymous heroine keeps the head of her dead lover in a pot of sweet basil, suggesting that it was indeed a herb used to mask the smell of deterioration. From *Isabella, or the Pot of Basil*:

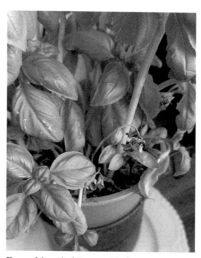

Potted basil. (*Emma Kay*)

> She wrapp'd it up; and for its tomb did choose
> A garden-pot, wherein she laid it by,
> And cover'd it with mould, and o'er it set
> Sweet Basil, which her tears kept ever wet.[103]

Belladonna: along with its witchy connotations; belladonna is both an opioid, which is basically a pain reliever, and an anti-spasmodic (decreasing muscle activity). Numerous experiments or cases of overdosing on belladonna by accident are recorded in literature across the centuries. In many instances the person consuming this herbaceous plant would end up paralysed for up to several days, often before making a full recovery. Paul Curie considered belladonna to be the only successful remedy for scarlet fever. He prescribed one to three 'globules' of belladonna to be dissolved in six spoonfuls of water and administered every hour.[104]

Betony: writing in the ninth century, Walafrid Strabo stressed the versatility of this herb which was equally effective fresh, dried, in a drink or fermented over time. He emphasized its capacity for healing wounds quickly when crushed directly over an injury.[105] Betony was utilized in abundance in ancient Egypt and Rome. Augustus Caesar's physician, Antonius Musa, wrote a whole manuscript about the benefits of betony, including its ability to cure headaches, as well as over forty other diseases. During the eighteenth century a company called Rowley's manufactured herb snuff which claimed to be:

> more efficacious in all Disorders of the Head and eyes, in strengthening the nerves and stomach, and in healing and comforting the Breast and Lungs, than anything of the kind ever yet dispensed. For besides the common ingredients of Betony, Coltsfoot, Eye-bright, Marum, Lavender, Thyme, Rosemary, there are several other medicinal Herbs, Woods, Barks, Gums &c. all approved Medicines …

The snuff was available to purchase from St. Paul's Coffee-House in London at a cost of two shillings and sixpence per cannister.[106]

Birthwort: I have read that birthwort was once considered a good antidote to scurvy back in the eighteenth century, while Greek, Roman and Byzantine physicians recommended it for a range of ailments from kidney disorders – ironically, large doses have proved to induce kidney poisoning and bladder stones – to gout and even for snakebites.[107] Medieval midwives considered birthwort to be an effective contraceptive; this was undoubtedly a consequence of its physical likeness to a womb or vagina, at a time when plants merely had to resemble a part of human anatomy to become synonymous with the healing of it.

Bistort: according to John Gerard, bistort had the power to secure loose teeth if held in the mouth around the tooth in question, at certain times of the day. He also advocated that if its juice were snorted, bistort could alleviate polyps in the nose.[108] It is also a herb that has been known to slow down the flow of internal bleeding. Bistort is a fairly powerful herb, which is largely taken for granted, perhaps due to the fact that it grows so abundantly. The root has been used on occasions to stem haemorrhaging and to relieve diarrhoea and dysentery.[109]

Borage was commonly consumed in the form of a distilled water. Both John Gerard and Nicholas Culpeper confirmed borage as a useful guard against madness. This was probably based on ancient definitions, such as Pliny's praise for the herb's ability to dispel melancholy. Bees are attracted to borage and as such it was often planted near hives to encourage the production of honey. With an aroma akin to cucumber borage gained a reputation as a refreshing and cleansing herb. In his *Earthly Paradise* John Parkinson commended its stunning blue flowers, which were eaten in salads in the Elizabethan era.[110]

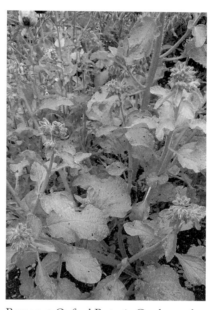

Borage at Oxford Botanic Garden and Arboretum. (*Emma Kay*)

Bryony (black): throughout the Middle Ages the root of black bryony was widely considered useful for healing rheumatic pains as a poultice. It was later exploited as a purgative by quacks. This could prove fatal due to its toxicity, as David Ellis notes in the 1918 edition of *Medicinal Herbs and Poisonous Plants*.[111] There are both white and black bryony. White bryony originally took the name of tetterberry, due to its healing abilities with a skin disease known as tetters, a vesicular condition such as eczema, herpes or ringworm. The root of bryony once held similar symbolic connotations to that of the mandrake, fashioned into the images of men, women or children and used as a magical talisman.[112]

Burdock or **Arctium** has had other names attached to it including cockle button hardock and beggars' buttons, but the word burdock derives from the French word for butter, *beurre*. This is because women in France would wrap their cakes of butter in the burdock leaves to keep them fresh in the heat while en route to market.[113] Burdock's enduring reputation of the past to remedy gout, sores and ulcers, among other things, meant it was commonly in use well into the twentieth century. Today, its roots still have a role as an antioxidant and it is used in a culinary capacity. Burdock was also the inspiration behind the invention of Velcro, with the ability of the natural hook system of its burs allowing it to attach themselves to fabric.

Caraway: this biennial plant was historically categorized as a herb by the Greek botanist Pedanius Discorides. Medicinally caraway is supposed to ease colic and flatulence and was often manufactured as an oil to be prescribed on a lump of sugar or in a teaspoon of hot water. The seeds are synonymous with a type of medieval confection called a comfit or added to cakes. The herb makes an appearance in William Shakespeare's *Henry IV*:

> Come, cousin silence! We will eat a pippin of last year's graffing, with a dish of Caraways, and then to bed!

As an earlier dish, the root of the caraway was integral to the Roman bread and milk pottage known as *chara*, alleged to have been eaten as warming, hearty fare for soldiers.[114]

Chives was also once known as *cepa* (Latin), rush-leeks, *cives* (old French), cyve and sweth amongst others. In the past there was confusion as to whether chives should fall under the category of onions or leeks, of which they are both related. Even Nicholas Culpeper was reluctant to add chives to his acclaimed *Complete Herbal* until he received a letter from someone who was able to persuade him of its legitimacy as a herb. Interestingly, Culpeper talks about the 'harmful vapours' they omitted which caused issues with eye sight. Not dissimilar to our all too familiar understanding of the chemical irritant syn-propanethial-S-oxide, which can make our eyes water when chopping onions. He also suggested eating them as a useful diueretic.[115] Chives were valued by the Romans and Marcus Valerius Martialis, a Roman satirist wrote:

He who bears chives on his breathe,
Is safe from being kissed to death.[116]

Along the line of Hadrian's Wall near Walltown in Northumbria, wild chives grow abundantly. The general consensus is that the presence of these chives is a consequence of Roman soldiers who cultivated various herbs and vegetables as they marched, to maintain a constant supply of medicinal plants. These chives may well be descendants of the Roman originals and they are now under a protection order.[117]

Calamint provides an ancient remedy for rheumatism, when bruised and applied directly to the skin.[118] Today it is the herb most associated with treating respiratory conditions. Calamint has a very pleasant, sweet aroma and delicate little white flowers which make nice cordials.

Chervil: with its faint taste of aniseed, chervil is used regularly in a culinary capacity, particularly in France. Saint Hildegard of Bingen considered this delicate parsley-like herb to be of considerable benefit to issues relating to the bowel if pounded down and mixed with wine. She also provides a method for making an ointment to treat ulcers of scabies by mixing chervil with ferns, cooking them in water, filtering the mixture, frying it in pork fat with frankincense and sulphur, before applying it to the skin and flesh over the course of five days.[119]

Chicory: there are numerous varieties of chicory with some traditionally being used as a substitute for coffee, others simply as salad leaves. Some old texts refer to varieties of chicory as endive; again there are different types of endive: French, Belgian, red, wild, witloof. In America, endive is more of a lettuce salad leaf. With so many different varieties and names it is often confusing to know which chicory was used for what purpose –or if endive was often just a generic name given to common chicory. Generally, this woody plant is today considered helpful

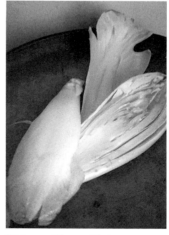

Chicory. (*Emma Kay*)

as a laxative and for conditions of the liver. The Victorians understood it to have 'an active influence upon the kidneys'; in other words, it was a good diuretic.[120] Chicory is also thought to increase appetite. John Gerard categorized 'Succorie' essentially as three separate plants: chicory/cichorie, endive and dandelion, with their own variants within this. He emphasized the common issue of confusing the different plants, which were often wrongfully lumped together. He believed that all variations were good for the liver, jaundice and as a sleep aid.[121]

Chamomile: Culpeper revered this herb, reminding his readers that the Egyptians deemed it a herb of the sun and as such it generates feelings of tremendous well-being. It acts as a mild sedative and is good for the digestion and as an anti-inflammatory. Known best for being taken in a tea, the flowers can also be added to warm baths to relieve general aches and pains as well as ground down to boost blond highlights in hair. Culpeper believed that if gall or kidney stones were removed from the body, they could 'dissolve' over time if wrapped in chamomile.[122] It would appear he wasn't the only one. There is actually a preparation for managing kidney and gall stones using chamomile that was published in the *Derby Mercury* in 1739. It goes like this:

> Take four ounces and a half of the best Alicant soap, beat it in a mortar with a large spoonful of swines-cresses [an English garden weed] burnt to a blackness, and as much Honey as will make the whole of the Consistence of Paste. Let this be form'd into a Ball. Take this Ball, and Green Chamomile or Chamomile Flowers, Sweet Fennel, Parsley and Burdock Leaves of each one ounce. When they are not Greens, take the same Quantities of roots, cut the Herbs or Roots, Slice the Ball, and boil them in two Quarts of soft Water half an Hour, then strain it off, and sweeten it with Honey.[123]

Colewort: as mentioned in the previous section, coleworts are many and varied. John Gerard meticulously discusses each of these in turn, but writes about their virtues generically. Mixed with fenugreek, he lists colewort as a remedy for gout, while noting its properties to alleviate canker sores around the eyes.[124]

Coltsfoot grows near water, its flowers are a vibrant yellow and its leaves, which famously appear after the flowers have died, have historically been smoked to aid catarrh and coughing since Grecian times. Its Latin name is *Tussilago farfara*, taken from *tussis ago*, or 'I drive away' (a cold). Coltsfoot comes with a health warning, as it can impact negatively on the liver, but it was once frequently administered as a treatment for whooping cough:

> Take of dried coltsfoot leaves, a good handful, cut them small and boil 'em in a pint of spring water till half a pint is boiled away; then take off fire, and when almost cold, squeezing the herbs as dry as you can, dissolve in the liquor an ounce of sugar candy, powdered, then give the child. One spoonful two to three times a day was the recommended dose for children aged 3–4, which was guaranteed to abate the coughing.[125]

Cowslips: now this is one I keep meaning to trial myself! A decoction made from the flowers of cowslips, as recommended by Nicholas Culpeper, could apparently 'taketh away spots and wrinkles of the skin, sun-burning and freckles, and adds beauty exceedingly'.[126]

Clary: this multi-functioning herb when mixed with wine allegedly becomes an aphrodisiac, while adding it to honey, clary can dissolve small ulcers that form in the corneas of eyes,[127] which dovetails with herbalist Maud Grieve's much later twentieth-century interpretation of clary as a useful eyewash.

Comfrey was frequently once referred to as 'boneset' and was grown in infirmary gardens for its abilities to heal wounds, and help heal broken bones and sprains. By the nineteenth century it was more popularly used as cattle feed. At one time comfrey, along with celandine and clover, if applied directly to the skin, professed to be useful at reducing visible tumours of a cancerous nature.

Coriander: it may be a surprise for some readers to learn that coriander is actually a herb and not a spice. In India coriander seeds are used to treat flatulence, as a diuretic and to improve digestion. They are also considered an aphrodisiac. The seeds are commonly used in pharmaceutical preparations to mask other powerful tastes or smells, or chewed to conceal halitosis.[128] In her *Curious Herbal*, Elizabeth Blackwell mentions that coriander was thought to help with the 'King's Evil' or scrofula, a form of tuberculous swelling of the lymph glands. Known as 'king's evil' throughout Europe for much of the medieval period, due to the fact that the royal touch was thought to cure this particular type of disease.[129]

Cress: John Gerard notes its many varieties and the fact that 'lowe countrie men', or the labouring classes, often ate cress with bread and butter, which I find ironic considering its association today with high teas and fancy sandwiches. He also mentions its abilities to prevent scurvy and when mixed with vinegar and barley it afforded a good remedy for sciatica.[130] In addition, John Parkinson noted the common prescription of cress seeds to children with parasitic worms.[131]

Dill: Hildegard's eleventh-century *Physica* cites dill as a herb, which when mixed with water, mint and other roots had the potential to prevent men from engaging in lustful thoughts. The mix required making into a vinegar to be taken daily with food.[132] Dill is mentioned in the bible as a herb that wasn't harvested like others using a threshing process; rather the plant was beaten until the seeds were released.

> When they have levelled its surface,
> do they not scatter dill, sow cummin,
> and plant wheat in rows
> and barley in its proper place,
> and spelt as the border?
>
> Dill is not threshed with a threshing-sledge,
> nor is a cartwheel rolled over cummin;
> but dill is beaten out with a stick,
> and cummin with a rod.[133]

By the nineteenth century this herb was regarded by some as beneficial to children, in particular for wind and gripe in babies.[134] Today dill is considered to be useful in the garden at eliminating slugs and moths.

Dittany: although there are several species, generically dittany is a plant which is native to Crete but grows throughout parts of Europe, Africa, Asia and even North America. It is a relative of marjoram and can be highly flammable in hot conditions and toxic; it can also give you a nasty stomach ache. John Parkinson wrote about its unusual abilities to remove dead foetuses from the womb, while other writers have praised the herb's capacity to heal wounds.[135]

Eyebright: it is understood that the pioneering early medieval German physician and alchemist Theophrastus von Hohenheim Paracelsus was responsible for introducing the world to the benefits of eyebright. Frequently promoted as a remedy for eye problems, this herbaceous flowering plant has a small black mark on each corolla, which quickly became associated with the pupil of an eye. Hence the tenuous relationship with optical care.[136] Culpeper suggested mixing distilled eyebright with wine or broth to help clear a person's vision. He also thought it could help stimulate memory.[137]

Feltwort: in addition to repelling unwanted beasts in its magical capacity, this hairy species of mullein was said to heal diarrhoea when the root was boiled in red wine and drunk. Boiled in water it could cure a continuous cough or internal cuts and abrasions, while eating the leaves or rubbing the affected area in the oil of the flowers shrank haemorrhoids apparently.[138]

Fennel: the early medieval abbotess, Hildegard of Bingen, rated fennel very highly as a medicinal herb. She believed that eating fennel or the seeds of fennel daily could rid a person of troublesome phlegm, bad breath and cloudy eyesight. She also had faith in its abilities to cure insomnia when mixed with other herbs, indigestion, melancholy and tumours among other ailments.[139] Chilblains were also frequently treated using a mix of fennel root, eggs and wine.

Garlic: in Sanskrit, the word garlic means 'slayer of monsters'. It gained the nickname 'poor man's treacle' at one time in England and was an antidote for animal poisons. In the county of Kent and perhaps other regions garlic was once placed in the stockings of children with whooping cough, as a cure. While in Cuba, thirteen cloves of garlic were worn around the neck for thirteen days to cure jaundice.[140] The ancient Egyptian papyrus *Ebers* suggests a poultice of rotten flesh, herbs of the field and garlic cooked in goose oil, taken over a period of four days to combat most physical weaknesses. Bulbs of garlic were also placed at the entrance of exposed holes to prevent snakes slithering out of them.[141]

Gentian: this powerful root, which is light brown in colour with a pungent, bitter taste, grows in abundance in the Alps and the Pyrenees and is named after the king of Illyria, Gentius. On the authority of the *Shen nong Ben cao jing*, the great Chinese book of medicinal plants and agriculture, this herb:

is bitter in flavour and cold … It is an important medicinal to drain fire from the liver and gallbladder. As such, it is able to brighten the eyes and cure jaundice caused by damp heat. Clinically, it is often used to treat fever, bone heat, abscesses and swellings, sores, scabs, roundworms, and, in children, fright epilepsy. It is also used for visiting hostility. This means a disease of sudden onset started by no identifiable cause and which is characterized by loss of consciousness, intense. fever, and/or delimits speech.[142.]

Hellebore: despite being a highly toxic plant, John Parkinson recommended white hellebore for dropsy, jaundice and a variety of ailments linked to the gall bladder and liver. The leaves or juice of the leaves along with the flowers could be fashioned into small cakes and baked, then eaten to treat the aforementioned.[143]

Henbane: writing in the twentieth century, pharmacologist David Macht noted that henbane or hebanon was once applied directly in the ear to ease earache during the Elizabethan era.[144] The ghost in *Hamlet* reveals the manner in which the king was murdered:

> Sleeping within mine orchard,
> My custom always of an afternoon,
> Upon my secure hour thine uncle stole,
> With juice of cursed hebanon in a phial,
> And in the porches of mine ears did pour
> The leprous distilment …[145]

Herb bennet or **avens**: allegedly, small quantities of the root of herb bennet were at one time added to ale to add flavour, in addition to its capacity for preventing the drink from going sour. The roots contain high levels of tannin, which made herb bennet integral to the trades of tanning leather and dyeing wool. By adding boiling water to the sliced root of this herb, it could be drunk to ease fevers, or utilized as a similar infusion for general stomach disorders, simply by adding syrup or ginger. Herb bennet was formerly esteemed for its antiseptic properties.[146]

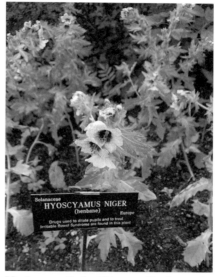

Henbane at Oxford Botanic Garden and Arboretum. (*Emma Kay*)

Herb robert is a member of the geranium family. It is that common weedlike flower that you will often find choking up your garden with its long stems and little pink flowers. In Tudor England it was one of the main herbs used as garden edgings; it also apparently made a very pleasant and warming tea. Pedanius Dioscorides recommended a teaspoonful mixed with wine to reduce any swellings of the vulva. He informs us in *De Materia Medica* that the Romans called it echinaster, while the African name is iesce.[147]

Horehound: there is white and black horehound. The former, which grows in abundance in Norfolk, was frequently used in remedies for asthma, coughs and as an expectorant. John Gerard suggested candying the leaves to relieve consumption. White horehound in milk was also believed to make an excellent fly killer. Black horehound leaves could be applied as a poultice to soothe gout.[148]

Hyssop: Avicenna's Islamic compendium, *Canon of Medicine*, prescribes hyssop mixed with maiden hair and cassia wood to rectify obstructions in the lungs.[149] Hyssop flowers were frequently worn by women in their hair, not only for their pleasing blue colour, but also for their strong aroma. It was added to broths and decoctions as a plant traditionally known for its antiseptic and expectorant qualities. Hyssop was a recognized protector against the evil eye and as such could once be found hanging up in people's houses.[150]

Juniper: according to Pedanius Dioscorides, juniper berries were integral to a special scent, invented by the Egyptians and used as an offering to the gods. *Cyphi*, as it was called, could be mixed into drinks to act as a generic antidote, as well as easing asthma. Other ingredients included olive oil, myrrh, raisins, cardamom and calamus.[151] *Aqua Vulneria* is a medieval concoction, which remained popular for several centuries, consisting of dried mint, the seeds and tops of angelica, wormwood, rosemary and oil of juniper which after being distilled was applied to a variety of wounds.[152]

Krameria root or **rhatany** is a South American shrub, the root of which was widely used throughout Europe and England in the nineteenth century. It is very astringent and woody, yet odourless and was used to ease diarrhoea and catarrh. Dentists have also been known to dilute a tincture of rhatany with water to make an astringent mouth wash. The following is a recipe to make a tincture for this very purpose:

Rhatany root in coarse powder form	2½ ounces
Proof spirit	1 pint

Macerate the rhatany root for forty-eight hours in fifteen fluid ounces of the spirit, in a closed vessel, agitating occasionally; then transfer to a percolator, and when the fluid ceases to pass, continue the percolation with the remaining five ounces of spirit. Afterwards subject the contents of the percolator to pressure, filter the product, mix the liquids, and add sufficient proof spirit to make one pint. Dose: ½ to 2 fluid drachms (1 drachm being equivalent to ⅛ of a fluid ounce).[153]

Lavender: writing in the eleventh century, Hildegard of Bingen documented the benefits of spike lavender which she suggested cooking in wine, with honey and water. According to Hildegard, drinking it warm could reduce pain in the liver and lungs.[154] Lavender has many modern associations with easing anxiety and alleviating insomnia. It has a long heritage of being used for medicinal purposes; as an oil it was designed to ease headaches, as a perfume to mask the smell of treatments and other medicines and as a cordial to aid indigestion, acid reflux or to revive a casualty of fainting.[155]

Lemon balm is sometimes called by its Greek name *melittena* or *bee balm*, as bees cling to it. It was introduced to Britain by the Romans. Dioscorides claimed that the leaves of this herb when added to wine could ease spider and dog bites. He also advocated its use as a mouth rinse for toothache and when added to salt it had the potential to dissolve certain types of tumours.[156]

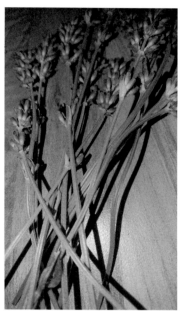

Lavender. (*Emma Kay*)

Liquorice (Glycyrrhiza glabra) is a perennial herb. John Gerard noted the power of liquorice root when used on sore throats, with its abilities to clear the passageways to the lungs. He praised its use as an expectorant and suggested, the trend at the time, adding it to gingerbread recipes. You can find an old recipe in Chapter 3. According to Gerard, sucking on liquorice could also quench your thirst. Liquorice was first cultivated around the time that Queen Elizabeth I came to the throne, particularly in the Pontefract area, unsurprisingly now home of the small, circular Pontefract liquorice cakes.

Lovage was once recognized as an emmenagogue herb, or a herb that is thought capable of stimulating menstrual flow. The seeds were used to combat flatulence, whereas an infusion of the root could help with kidney stones and even jaundice.[157] Many of these recommendations, outlined in the Victorian era, are an exact echo of Pedanios Dioscorides's pharmacopeia *De Materia Medica* written in circa 50 AD.

Marshmallow: the twelfth-century compendium *Trotula*, named after its assumed female writer Trota of Salerno, recommended the following concoction for children born with one limb larger than the other:

... bear's breech (Acanthus mollis) with root of marshmallow and with leaves of wild celery, parsley and fennel, and all diuretic herbs. Boil these in water. And let the limb of the patient be placed above the vessel, and let it be covered with a linen cloth so that it sweats. Then let chamomile and marshmallow be cooked in water, and in this thick mixture let wax be melted, and let the whole limb then be covered with this. Afterward, let it be tied tightly with linen bandages, and thus let the limb of the patient sweat through one night; in the morning, let it be rubbed so that the spirits are aroused and flow to the painful part.

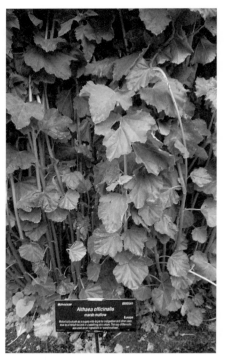

Marshmallow at Oxford Botanic Garden and Arboretum. (*Emma Kay*)

There is more rubbing and anointing and more cooking of marshmallow before bandaging the whole limb, which needed to be rested, with the patient receiving regular quantities of red wine. It is emphasized by the writer, that this procedure will only work on a very recent affliction.[158]

Marjoram: as stated by Scottish physician Thomas Short, wild marjoram was best infused in a tea to alleviate asthma, coughing and difficulties with digestion. He also praised its potential for curing the hiccups, when blended with cloves and sugar.[159] As a herbal remedy today marjoram is still considered beneficial to coughs, colds and indigestion. According to Rosalind Northcote, the scent of marjoram used to be very highly prized. The medieval herbalist John Parkinson is said to have recorded it was a herb 'put in nosegays, and in the windows of houses, as also in sweete pouders, sweete bags, and sweete washing waters ... Our daintiest women doe put it to still among their sweet herbes'. Unsurprisingly, marjoram was a popular herb for strewing.[160]

Milk thistle is so called for its leaves were said to mimic the colour of the Virgin Mary's milk which spilled onto the plant while Mary was breastfeeding Jesus. The seeds, or more specifically the membrane covering the seeds of this plant, were believed to help with obstructions in the liver and for jaundice. Pedanius Dioscorides asserted its abilities to encourage vomiting when drunk together with honey.[161]

Mint: the ancient Egyptians suggested rubbing peppermint all over the bottom to induce labour and to 'protect against everything' (quite a claim); the scrapings of a statue, along with wild mint, cooked together in oil and wax was recommended.[162] According to Pliny several measures of mint, with a single measure of sulphur, beaten with vinegar or vinegar and soot could provide a useful remedy for the skin disorder, erysipelas.[163] Dioscorides believed mint to be an aphrodisiac as well as preventing milk from curdling. He also acknowledged its benefits to the stomach and culinary prowess as a good sauce. [164]

Naulewort or **pennywort** has several varieties. Wall pennywort (navelwort) was understood to alleviate chapped heels, which required bathing before the leaves were applied over the dry area.
The leaves and roots were also administered to remedy dropsy, a term for swelling caused by water retention.[165] Today pennywort is sometimes used in the treatment of earache in herbal medicine.

Nettles: Culpeper wrote at length about the medicinal benefits of nettles. The roots or leaves boiled in juice then mixed with honey and sugar was recommended as a means of clearing the lungs and curing shortness of breath. Both the leaves or seeds of nettles were also used to expel gall and kidney stones as well as kill tapeworms in children. A distilled water made from nettles according to Culpeper also helped alleviate 'morphew', when the skin was cleansed in it. Morphew is an old name for scurvy and leprosy. A simple handful of nettles, together with wallwort/danewort, gently bruised and applied to gout or sciatica could soothe away all the associated aches and pains.[166] Culpeper's claims relating to worms is an interesting one when you consider that in the 1990s and maybe still today, communities living in the Kashmir Himalayas traditionally suffered from extreme worm infestations as a consequence of poor sanitation. Every

September the people of the Karnah valley collected nettle roots in large quantities, washed and dried them thoroughly before boiling them in water for up to three hours. Patients suffering from worms were then given this to drink once a week, which was said to bring great relief.[167]

Oregano: Trota's twelfth-century compendium of women's medicine suggests bathing in a treatment of pennyroyal, oregano, catmint, laurel and marshmallow to cure pains in the womb.[168] Oregano is a staple of Mexican cooking.

Paris quadrifolia: the plant herb 'true love' or true lover's knot, now known as Paris quadrifolia, was considered magical due to its four leaves which are arranged as opposing pairs. As such it gained the reputation for effectively being able to break a spell that had enchanted someone.[169] Chaucer mentions Paris quadrifolia in his *Miller's Tale*. He refers to it as the 'trewelove' herb, suggesting it provided a combination of both aphrodisiac and piety:

> Whan that the firste cok hath crowe, anon
> Up rist this joly lovere Absolon,
> And him arraieth gay, at point-devis.
> But first he cheweth geyn and licoris,
> To smellen sweete, er he hadde kiembd his heer.
> Under his tonge a trewe-love he beer,
> For therby wende he to ben gracious.[170]

Parsley: Bald's early medieval text, the *Leechbook*, suggests coriander and parsley kneaded into bread or rubbed into wine as a remedy for issues relating to the spleen, while Dioscorides writing around AD 60, considered common garden parsley as an excellent curative for menstrual issues.[171]

Pennyroyal: Walafrid Strabo, the German Benedictine monk, regarded this herb as the greatest of all in terms of its many virtues, although he scorned its exploitation by others, as a cure-all herb. Strabo declared that it could revive a 'sluggish stomach', with the use of a poultice or in a drink. Despite his logical mind he also wrote:

'If you stick a twig of pennyroyal behind your ear, then the sun's heat won't make you dizzy when it beats down upon you in the open.'[72]

Radish was viewed as both herb and vegetable in medieval England. It is another of the country's oldest edible roots with a recorded legacy dating back to circa 300 BC. Gervase Markham prized it for its ability to soothe 'cloyed stomacks' and for its capacity to grow easily and abundantly from seed. In the ninth century, Walafrid Strabo claimed it was a cure for violent coughing.[173]

Rosemary: the virtues of rosemary are varied. It is perhaps best known for strengthening the memory and in some parts of Greece, older members of the community infuse water with rosemary and use it to wash their hair.[174] I'm wondering if this tradition has as much to do with infusing the head and mind, as well as providing an aromatic shampoo. Pliny believed that the fresh roots of rosemary could heal wounds and ease haemorrhoids, while the seed when mixed with wine and pepper could help with urinary disorders. He also thought it was possible to remove skin freckles by applying rosemary.[175] Elizabeth Blackwell noted rosemary's abilities to assist with troubles relating to the

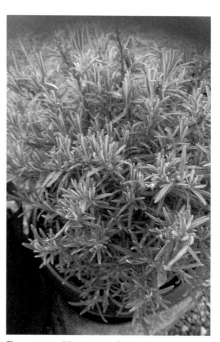

Rosemary. (*Emma Kay*)

head and nerves, as well as to sweeten the air while improving memory and sight.[176] The notion of rosemary as a protection against putrid smells is evident in Thomas Dekker's account of the plague in 1603, noting 'the price of flowers, hearbes and garlands rose wonderfully, in so much that Rosemary which had wont to be sold for 12 pence and armful, went now for six shillings a handfull'.[177] (See Chapter 3 for bread fritters recipe and more about this fascinating herb.)

Ragwort: John Gerard noted its regular use by physicians in the seventeenth century on 'greene wounds' and old ulcers. It was an early remedy for arthritis and rheumatism when mixed together with pig's fat to form an ointment, in addition to relieving sciatica if blended with frankincense and mastic oil.[178]

Rue: Walafrid Strabo compiled the hugely important ninth-century horticultural document, *Hortulus*. This volume records the medieval monastic garden that he tended in great detail. He describes rue as powerfully fragrant, with the ability to relieve 'hidden toxins and expel harmful substances from their troubled bowels'.[179] In recent years rue has been studied for its positive effects on epilepsy, which, according to Fard and Shojaii in 2013 has more of an ability to delay a seizure, rather than manage it.[180] A few sprigs of rue are still added to bottles of the Greek alcoholic drink tsipouro, or raki, as it is thought to cleanse the blood. Rue is also understood to act as a useful insect repellent.[181]

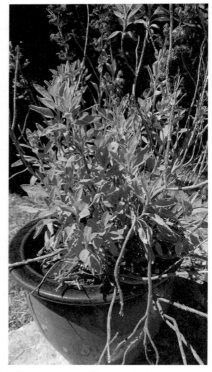

Sage has an established reputation for its abilities to enhance memory. Roman author and naturalist Pliny and Greek philosopher Celsus maintained that sage could cure symptoms of the plague, as well as kill worms and restore a person's memory. It was also boiled together with wine, rosemary (another herb linked to memory), honeysuckle and plantain to sooth a sore throat.[182] Recent clinical trials on the benefits of sage with recalling memory have yielded positive outcomes. In 2003 the Medicinal Plant Research Centre (MPRC) at the Universities of Newcastle and Northumbria tested forty-four young adults using sage or a placebo. Following a word recall test, those who took the sage oil consistently demonstrated far greater results and

Flowering sage. (*Emma Kay*)

the herb is currently being investigated for the potential treatment of Alzheimer's disease.[183] Apparently, memory and sore throats have not been the only thing historically to benefit from sage. Samuel Pepys had no children and he mentions in his diaries about consulting with a man for advice about fertility during a dinner party. The guidance he was given included drinking the juice of sage.[184]

Savin: a mixture of the oil of savin and verdigris (the greenish powder formed on copper and brass after exposure to water) was used with some frequency in the Victorian period to remove venereal warts.[185] Interestingly, the first-century Greek physician Dioscorides claimed that savin was a herb with the potential to dissolve carbuncles, which mirrors the Victorian understanding of this needle-like leafed shrub.[186]

Savory: the eleventh-century botanist Hildegard of Bingen believed that savory could ease anxiety and lift a person's mood.[187] Culpeper valued it highly as a herb everyone should have around, preferably made into conserves and syrups for blocked bowels and cholic. He also recommended savory heated with rose oil and dropped into the ears to cure tinnitus.[188]

Senna has long been recognized for its purgative abilities, most obviously perhaps as a relief for constipation. It has a slightly unpleasant aroma and a bitter taste.[189]

Sorrel: while Hildegard of Bingen understood sorrel to be a herb that could stimulate depression when eaten. John Gerard thought it worked well in sauces that accompanied meats, in addition to being beneficial to the stomach when made into the equivalent of a spinach tart.[190]

St. John's Wort is widely known for its abilities to relieve anxiety and depression. It is also associated with antibacterial properties and for fighting skin irritations. It is still revered in most Greek households and is added to olive oil or infused in tea to heal cuts.[191]

Tarragon: John Parkinson wrote about the common misconception of tarragon as a herb that was cultivated by placing flax seeds into the root of an onion, a notion that he deemed 'absurd'. John Evelyn said of tarragon:

'Tis highly cordial and friend to the head, heart and liver.'[192] Tarragon was a herb that was used in conjunction with other 'cold' herbs to counteract heat and one more typically used in salads in medieval times, rather than medicinally.[193]

Thyme: according to Lemery, writing in 1745, thyme stimulates the brain. It was also said to arouse appetite. Undoubtedly these theories probably stem from its agreeable and aromatic smell.[194] It was categorized as hot and dry and was known to be good for the uterus and for prompting women's monthly menstrual cycles. Most interestingly of all is a recipe in which thyme played the central role when infused with rose wine and oil of 'saffafras', which is probably a misspelling of the flowers, roots or bark of the sassafras tree, a species of North American and Asian trees which are nearly all but extinct. This concoction was said to cure the green sickness.[195] Green sickness or 'the disease of virgins', is the historical term for a type of anaemia. Identified by the English physician Johannes Lange in 1554, it was originally attributed to pubescent girls who failed to menstruate, combined with a greenish pallor and eating disorders. Defining the meaning of this illness has fluctuated over the centuries and its social context has changed. A real diagnosis of the green sickness remains debateable.[196] Incidentally, sassafras is still said to be used in the production of America's iconic root beer beverage.

Vervain or **verbena** is odourless and tasteless and was typically made into amulets or included in sacrificial rites, before becoming more recognized for its genuine medicinal properties. Vervain worked best worn around the neck to cure headaches. Over the years verbena has been associated with all manner of beneficial treatments; in the form of eye ointments, as a cure for ulcers and as an uplifting herb it is capable of inspiriting when added to drinking water.[197]

Wormwood is a bitter herb, which in Anglo-Saxon times was taken as a cordial to expel a fever. It was also boiled up and poured over the head to relieve dizziness and headaches.[198] In Moroccan folk medicine, wormwood is used to treat high blood pressure and diabetes.[199]

Yarrow: the preface to hops was yarrow, with the leaves and flowers once widely used to flavour beer. It can halt the flow of blood and as such became synonymous with treating heavy menstruation. Yarrow is also an antibiotic and antiseptic thanks to its menthol, insulin, quercetin, camphor and salicylic makeup.[200] As a very early treatment this herb was used to cure hiccups. The root of the yarrow needed to be pounded down and mixed with beer, which had to be drunk lukewarm.[201]

Chapter 3

Culinary Transition

'A Man may esteem himself happy when that which is his food is also his medicine.'[1]

Undoubtedly the use of herbs in contemporary multicultural British society has altered considerably in the last century. As immigration has risen, so too has the demand for a broader variety of herbs. Southern Asian communities require more coriander and parsley, Turkish communities oregano and mint, while basil and rosemary are staples of Southern European cuisine.

Today Britain imports most of its more exotic herbs from Antarctica, which are cultivated in huge greenhouses designed to supply isolated crews with fresh vegetables. The UK also imports herbs from Bhutan in South Asia, the East African coast, Central Africa and Madagascar.

The way we prepare herbs compared to the past also differs. By 1900, most cooks were already using dried instead of fresh herbs. It was once

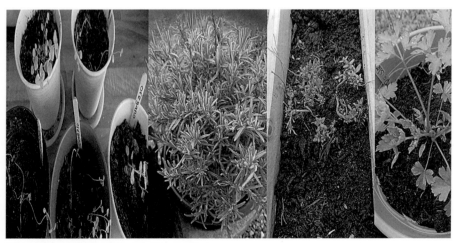

Mixed Mediterranean herbs. (*Emma Kay*)

common practice for herbs to be grown at home in the garden, picked fresh for every new dish. The 1631 edition of Markham's *English House-Wife* provides detailed advice on the cultivation and use of culinary herbs and while there has undeniably been an increase in recent years for individual households to grow more of their own vegetables, fruit and herbs; gone are the days of the mandatory traditional kitchen garden.

With Chapter 1 focusing predominantly on white, British herbalists and botanists, this chapter includes a variety of global historic recipes that rely on herbs. Some have been translated, others updated for the modern cook.

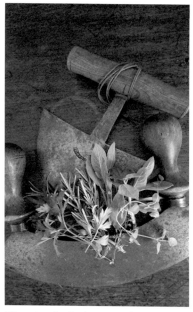

Victorian herb choppers. (*Emma Kay*)

Soups and Stews

In medieval Britain soups were known generally as pottages (in the pot), consisting mostly of vegetables and oats which were flavoured with herbs. Wealthier communities had access to exotic imported spices and more meat, which enhanced their diet. The fourteenth-century naturalist Henry Daniel noted that chervil, borage, mallows, three sorts of orach (eaten as spinach) and turnip roots were very good ingredients for pottages.[2]

Herb bennet which is short for St. Benedict and is also sometimes called wood avens or colewort, is cited in the subsequent recipe. It was once a favoured seasoning of the British Isles, with the Romans using it as an alternative to quinine. (See Chapter 2 for its association with witchcraft.) The following method of making vegetable stew is taken from *The Forme of Cury* which is the collective term for six manuscripts now widely considered to represent the first English cookbook. Dating to the late fourteenth century and recognized as the work of authors who cooked for King Richard II, it covers a variety of dishes from extravagant feasts to everyday fare. *The Forme of Cury* includes recipes that incorporate a number of rare, luxury imports such as cinnamon, ginger and nutmeg, as well as the proficient use of sugar.

Outes/Eowtes
Take Borage, cool. Langdebef. Persel. Betes orage auance. violet. saueray. and fenkel. and whane þey buth sode; presse hem wel smale. cast hem in gode broth an seeþ hem. and serue hem forth.

Vegetable stew (my translation)
Take borage, colewort, langdebeef (or bristly oxtongue, a type of daisy), beets, herb bennet, violet leaves, savory and fennel. And when they have boiled, crush them down and add them to a good broth.[3]

Fennel is one of England's oldest established herbs and has long been used in cooking; along with its relative, which is considered more of a vegetable, Florence fennel. Both add a characteristic aniseed flavour to a variety of dishes. As the following recipe calls for sliced 'blades', I am assuming that it is referring to the cut bulb more akin to the Florence variety.

Fenkel in Soppes
(A dish consisting of a soup or broth poured over a slice of toasted bread.) Take blades of Fenkel. shrede hem not to smale, do hem to seeþ in water and oile and oynouns mynced þerwith. do þerto safroun and salt and powdour douce, serue it forth, take brede ytosted and lay the sewe onoward.

Fennel broth on toast (my translation)
Slice the fennel bulb. Soak the slices in water, oil, and minced onions. Add saffron and salt to taste. Take some toasted bread and spread the mixture on top.[4]

Jowtes or joutes was a soup of either boiled vegetables or pot herbs. Sometimes this dish was thickened with breadcrumbs or it was added to other broths or almond milk. Joutes was a popular dish that also appears in the fourteenth-century epic poem, *Piers Plowman*:

> I have be cook in hir kichene,
> And the covent served
> Manye monthes with hem,

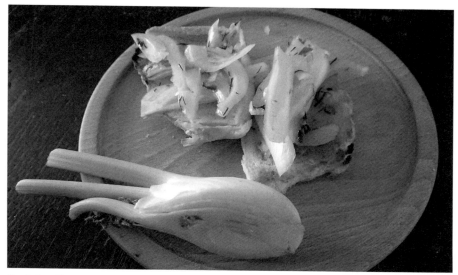

Fenkel in Soppes. (*Emma Kay*)

> And with monkes bothe.
> I was the prioresse potager,
> And othere povere ladies,
> And maad hem joutes of janglyng …[5]

Joutes also feature in *The Forme of Cury*

Jowtes of almaund mylke

Take erbes, boile hem, hewe hem and grynde hem smale. and drawe hem up with water. set hem on the fire and seeþ the rowtes with the mylke. and cast þeron sugur & salt. & serue it forth.[6]

Joutes in almond milk (my translation)

Take a good handful of pot herbs, such as borage, parsley, beet leaves and leeks. Slice and dice them. Wash and drain them in a cloth and soak the joutes in enough almond milk to cover them before heating and simmering. Add sugar and salt to taste. Serve.

A composte was a compote, a dish soaked in liquid, a compounded mix of many ingredients, basically another word used for an early stew. This recipe for a chicken compote contains lovage, which has a very distinctive flavour that is likely to overpower most dishes. Today it is recognized for its potential in the treatment of inflammation and as a mild sedative.

The following recipe appears in the English cookbook of 1430, *Liber Cure Cocorum*. Much of the text is written in a specific northern dialect and as such, it is frequently attributed to Lancashire.

For to make a compost

> Take þo chekyns and hew hom for þo seke,
> All but þe hede and þe legges eke;
> Take a handfulle of herb lovache,
> And anoþer of persely, als
> Of sage þat never was founde fals,
> And noþer of lekes and alle hom wasshe
> Þose herbes in water, þat rennes so rasshe;
> Breke þorowghe þy honde, bothe herbe and leke,
> With a pynt of hony enbeny hom eke,
> Summe of þese herbes þou shalle laye
> In þe pottus bothun, as I þe say;
> Summe of þe chekyns þou put þerto,
> And þen of þe herb3 do to also;
> So of þo ton so of þat oþer,
> Þo herb3 on þe last my dere brother;
> Above þese herbus a lytul larde
> Smalle myncyd, haldand togeder warde;
> Take powder of gynger and canel god wone,
> Cast on þese oþer thynges everychon;
> Be sle3e and powre in water þenne
> To myd þo pot, as I þe kenne;
> Opone þo bruys poure hit withinne,
> And cover hit þat no hete oute wynne,
> And tendurly seyth hit þou do may,
> Salt hit, serve hit, as I þe say.[7]

For to make a compote (my translation)

> Take the chickens and chop them small enough for the stewing pan,
> All but the head and the legs also;
> Take a handful of the herb lovage,

And another of parsley, also
Of sage that was never found false,
And another of leeks and
wash all the herbs in water;
Crush the herbs and leeks with your hands,
Baste them with a pint of honey also,
Lay some of the herbs in the bottom of the pot.
Add some of the chickens and then the herbs, then repeat
one after the other,
finishing with a layer of herbs;
Add a little lard.
Take powder of ginger and cinnamon [a] good quantity,
cover with water.
And cover the pan so that no heat comes out,
boil it gently.
Salt it, serve it.

Giblet soup

Take three sets of goose giblets, cleaned, cut into pieces, and blanched, add to them a small quantity of knotted marjoram [there are two types of marjoram – knotted and sweet], savory, thymes, basil, and parsley chopt fine; likewise four large onions, peeled and chopt, with eight escahllots [shallots], a little beaten spices, pepper and salt, and two quarts of water; when the giblets are three parts done, pick them from the herbs, and chop the bones down; put the giblets into a pot with boiled eggs and forcemeat balls; strain the liquor, let it settle, have ready three ounces of fresh butter and four passed over a fire for five minutes, then add to it half a pint of madeira or sherry wine, the liquor of the giblets, free from sediment, juice of lemon, cayenne pepper, and salt to the palate, and two quarts of good beef broth; make it boil, add to the giblets; let them stew gently till tender, and skim clean from fat.[8]

Nigerian herbs are used in cooking, as much as they are in medical applications. Bitter leaf or *Vernonia amygdalina*, so called due to the tart taste, is harvested in Nigeria from shrubs, and is used fresh or dried to enhance soups, eaten as a vegetable, or made into herbal infusions to treat anything from nausea to breast cancer.

The Nigerian herb beletientien is very similar to tarragon and is added to a variety of regional dishes, particularly in a traditional palm fruit pulp called banga. Another historically conventional ingredient of banga was African Lemongrass, known for its abilities to relive stress and promote sleep. It is also an antioxidant and can strengthen the immune system as well as being used to relieve thrush and yeast infections.

The following recipe for banga has been taken from the *Nigerian Cookbook*, containing both beletientien and lemongrass.

Banga (palm fruit pulp) soup with beef

1kg of palm fruit pulp from palm nuts
450g of beef pieces
1 tsp dry ground red pepper
½ a small onion
1 dstspn tomato paste
4 atarodo (or scotch bonnet) peppers
6 small okra
You may wish to add ½ tsp of atariko, ½ tsp of rigije, a blade of lemongrass and/or 1dstspn of beletientien to the pulp
Salt to taste

Make the strained fruit pulp up to 500ml of water and put in a pot with the meat. Boil on a low heat until tender. Grind the onion and fresh pepper and chop the okra finely. Add to the meat with the remaining ingredients and cook rapidly for 15 minutes, uncovered. The final cooking is best done in a local clay cooking pot as the liquid evaporates more quickly, resulting in a thicker soup without prolonged cooking. Served with pounded yam, cooked casava starch or tuwo (cooked rice or maize millet).[9]

The fourteenth-century cookbook *Le Viandier de Taillevent* or *Taillevant's, The Food Provider*, is commonly attributed to Guillaume Tirel; also known as Taillevant, a pioneering French cook, who trained as a young boy in the kitchens of Charles IV, rising in rank to serve Charles V, before attaining the title of master of the king's kitchen to Charles VI. He lived an extraordinarily long life for the period, dying at around the age of 80. The engraving on his tombstone depicts him with a shield illustrated with three stew-pots. While general consumers today tend to crave the main four big herbs often associated with French cooking – chives, parsley, tarragon and chervil – *Le Viandier* appears to only include parsley out of this super group of herbs. According to the text, herbs used to enhance the colour green in cooking during the 1300s included parsley, avens (gardenia), sorrel, gooseberries, vine leaves and green wheat; while it would appear spices were much more in fashion to flavour food during this period, in particular: ginger, cinnamon, cloves, grains of paradise (Guinea pepper), long pepper, round pepper, cinnamon flowers, saffron, nutmeg and cumin. Thyme and spike lavender were used a little and of course, garlic.

Green egg and cheese soup

Take parsley, a bit of sage, just a bit of saffron in the greens, and soaked bread, and steep in puree [of peas] or boiled water. Add ginger steeped in wine, and boil. Add the cheese, and the eggs when they have been poached in water. It should be thick and bright green. Some do not add bread, but add almond milk.[10]

Salads

Green, leafy salads, tossed in oil or vinegars have a heritage that extends to early Greek, Roman and Arabic cultures, while during the Middle Ages in England they often consisted of cooked vegetables with a selection of herbs. By the nineteenth century all manner of specialist salads emerged, including the Waldorf salad, Salade niçoise, potato salad (which is actually based on the Japanese dish Potesara), egg salad and of course the Caesar salad at the beginning of the twentieth century. There are hundreds of salads today, spanning many cultures and containing diverse ingredients.

Salat

Take persel, sawge, garlec, chibolles, oynouns, leek, borage, myntes, porrectes , fenel and ton tressis, rew, rosemarye, purslarye, laue and waische hem clene, pike hem, pluk hem small wiþ þyn honde and myng hem wel with rawe oile. lay on vynegur and salt, and serue it forth.[11]

Salad (my translation)

Take parsley, sage, garlic, spring onions, leek, borage, mint, young leeks, fennel and cress, rue, rosemary and purslane. Wash them clean and break them down into small pieces with your hands. Add oil, vinegar and salt and serve.

The sharp-tasting herb sorrel was once often eaten in salads and sauces. According to John Gerard, sorrel was a very popular herb in medieval sauces paired with various meats, particularly in the summer months.[12] The leaves of sorrel were also added to ale, or mixed into a posset as a means of quenching thirst and relieving the symptoms of pestilent fever, like the bubonic plague. [13]

The following recipe is for a warm salad which includes all manner of herbs including sorrel. It is taken from John Murrell's *A New Booke of Cookerie*, London, 1615:

Diuers Sallets boyled (a different boiled salad)

PArboyle Spinage, and chop it fine,
with the edges of two hard Trenchers
vpon a boord, or the backe of two
chopping Kniues: then set them on a
Chafingdish of coales with Butter and
Uinegar. Season it with Sinamon,
Ginger, Sugar, and a few parboyld
Currins. Then cut hard Egges into
quarters to garnish it withall, and serue
it vpon sippets. So may you serue
Burrage, Buglosse, Endiffe, Suckory,
Coleflowers, Sorrel, Marigold leaues,
water-Cresses, Leekes boyled, Onions,
Sparragus, Rocket, Alexanders. Parboyle
them, and season them all alike:
whether it be with Oyle and Uinegar,
or Butter and Uinegar, Sinamon,
Ginger, Sugar, and Butter: Egges
are necessary, or at least very good for
all boyld Sallets.[14]

The Russian household instruction manual of the sixteenth century. *The Domostroi*, compiled under the reign of the first tsar, better known as Ivan the Terrible, is one of the oldest known cookery books to emerge from this country. It mentions the use of herbs in cooking and in sorcery, which was strictly forbidden.

Perhaps the most iconic of Russian culinary manuals is Elena Molokhovets's *Classic Russian Cooking: A Gift to Young Housewives*, first published in 1861. Elena was to Russia what Isabella Beeton became to England or Fanny Farmer to the United States. Dill, chervil, tarragon and parsley form the historical backbone of Russian cooking, with dill even added to communion wine. All four of these herbs can be found in one of Elena Molokhovets's recipes for salad to accompany fish:

Elena Molokhovets's salad for fish

Slice green beans evenly and boil them in salted water until tender. When cooked, turn them into a colander, rinse with cold water, and set them on ice. In exactly the same manner boil asparagus, potatoes, and cauliflower. After they have been rinsed with cold water, mix them with the beans. Also add fresh peeled cucumbers, baked beets (all of these sliced or cut into pieces), parsley, dill, tarragon and chervil. Season with 2–3 spoons vinegar, olive oil, salt, a little mustard and sugar.[15]

English cookery author, Eliza Acton, writing about salads in her book of 1845, *Modern Cookery in all its Branches*, noted:

> The herbs and vegetables for a salad cannot be too freshly gathered; they should be carefully cleared from insects and washed with scrupulous nicety; they are better when not prepared until near the time of sending them to table, and should not be sauced until the instant before they are served. Tender lettuces, of which the outer leaves should be stripped away, mustard and cress, young radishes, and occasionally chives or small green onions … are the usual ingredients of summer salads.

And here is Eliza's recipe for French salad.

French salad
In winter this is made principally of beautifully blanched endive, washed delicately clean and broken into small branches with the fingers, then taken from the water and shaken dry in a basket kept for the purpose, or in a fine cloth; then arranged in the salad bowl, and strewed with herbs (tarragon generally, when in season) minced small.[16]

Sauces

Chinese soybean paste which was referenced in the second-century text, *The Rites of Zhou*, is probably the earliest reference to a sauce of sorts. French culinary historian and chef Henri Lecourt wrote an in-depth investigation of Chinese cooking in the 1920s, including an ancient recipe for soybean paste. Translated, it reads :

Puree soy
Cook four pieces of soybeans in water, put them in a cloth and squeeze them to extract the water. Throw this paste into two ounces of hot lard and add three ounces of soy-seasoned cucumbers and two ounces of soy ginger, all very finely chopped. Mix with a spinner and serve in a dish after drizzling with a tenth of an ounce of sesame oil.[17]

The French word *sauce* comes from the Latin *salsa*, meaning salted. One of the oldest European sauces which was hugely popular across the Roman empire was garum, or fish sauce; but verjuice or vinegar, once made primarily from sorrel, was undoubtedly also introduced to Britain by the Romans. Later it became the product of unripe fruit that was pressed and then preserved on the basis of its high acidity, opposed to using fermentation. Verjuice was used extensively in cooking throughout the sixteenth and seventeenth centuries. In his *Country Housewife and Lady's Director* of 1736, Richard Bradley, who was also a renowned botanist, recommended making verjuice from grapes, rather than crab apples, for a richer outcome. He also noted that crab apple verjuice was routinely applied to the art of calico printing. One thing we tend to overlook is the extent with which early medieval England cultivated vineyards and the amount of grapes that were once produced for all manner of purposes. Incidentally, the medieval German version of verjuice was called Agraz, using both grapes and apples, which is actually named after the South American wild blueberry.[18]

Verjuice (vinegar)

Take grapes full grown, just before they begin to ripen, and bruise them, without the trouble of picking them from the bunches; then put them in a bag, made of horse-hair and press them till the juice is discharged; put this liquor into a stone jar, leaving it uncovered for some days, then close it and keep it for use. N.B. It will do well, if the liquor is put into common casks, but is nicer to the palate if it is kept in glazed jars of about eight or nine gallons, and the berries might then be picked from the stalks.[19]

Verjuice in Britain was generally used as a sort of base sauce, which was added to others, including all types of what were generically known as 'green sauces'. These were typically made with spinach, or a variety of herbs like chervil and parsley, anything that was green basically. Another sauce similar to green sauce was the French sauce piquant, regularly an accompaniment to cold meats.

Sauce piquant (a sharp or relishing sauce)

Soak a good slice of veal and ham; when it catches, add a glass of white wine, half a glass of vinegar, two spoonfuls of broth, two of oil, two cloves of garlic, two slices of peeled lemon, a little tarragon, a laurel leaf, one of mint, two cloves, a little coriander; boil for an hour on a slow fire, reduce it to the consistency of a sauce, skim the fat very clean, and sift it in a sieve, you may add a little cullis, if you would have it thicker.[20]

Chasseur or 'hunter's sauce', due to its historical pairing with game meats is most associated with its origins in French cuisine. Charles Herman Senn was a Swiss cook and prolific culinary author of the past, who remains shamefully overlooked today. His *Book of Sauces* is one of my most prized gastronomical reference books and it contains several incredible variations of chasseur sauce, along with a standard game sauce, which is too marvellous to omit. It is also packed full of herbs.

Trained by Francatelli, consultant to the National Training School for Cookery and integral member of the Universal Cookery and Food Association, which evolved into the current Craft Guild of Chefs, Senn died at his desk in London, twenty years after his *Book of Sauces*, in collaboration with Brown and Polson, was heralded as the most complete volume of sauce recipes in the world.[21]

So, without further ado, here is Senn's marvellous game sauce or sauce gibier. For those unfamiliar with espagnole sauce (Spanish sauce), this is a classic French staple, a base or foundation sauce, made from roasted meat bones, sugar herbs and spices and tomato puree.

Game sauce

Some game bones and trimmings, 1 pint espagnole sauce or brown sauce, ½ gill sherry, onion, carrot, turnip, parsley, thyme, marjoram, bay-leaf, mace, clove.

The trimmings, carcasses, etc, of any kind of game may be used for this sauce; those of grouse or woodcock are preferable. Chope small the trimmings of game, put them in a stewpan with a small onion, a piece of carrot, and a piece of turnip all cut in slices, a few sprigs of parsley, a sprig of thyme, one of marjoram, a bay-leaf, a small piece of mace, and one clove, moisten with the sherry, cover, and put on the fire to cook for five minutes. Now add the espagnole or brown sauce, let it come quickly to a boil, and keep simmering for fifteen minutes longer. Pass through a tammy cloth, return to a clean stew-pan, season with a little salt if necessary, and keep hot in the bain-maries until required for serving.[22]

Vinegars, like sauces were once many and varied and carefully chosen to accompany the richness of game, to add flavour to fish, substance to pies or sweetness to desserts. Herbs and spices would have been integral to this process.

Tarragon vinegar

Pick the leaves off the stalks of green tarragon, just before it goes into bloom, and put a pound weight of every gallon of white wine vinegar, and treat it in the same manner as elder vinegar.

Glasse recommends the following for elder vinegar:

Let [it] steep and stir every day for a fortnight; then strain the vinegar from the flowers, press them close and let it stand to settle; then pour it from the settlings and put a piece of filtering paper in a funnel, and filter it through; then put it in pint bottles, cork it close, and keep it for use.[23]

Throughout Europe, early medieval sauces varied from both light, herb, pepper, or butter based, to heavily spiced sauces made with eggs. This one from fourteenth-century Germany, called Swallenberg, even contains honey, a throwback to Roman times:

Swallenberg sauce
Take wine and honey. Set that on the fire and let it boil. And add thereto pounded ginger more than pepper. Pound garlic, but not all too much, and make it strong and give it impetus with egg whites. Let it boil until it begins to become brown. One should eat this in cold weather.[24]

Vegetable Dishes

Historically the distinction between vegetables and some herbs has always been marginal, with herbs as a subset of their more substantial and less strongly flavoured relatives. As such, some main vegetable dishes were simply an arrangement of large leafy herbs – or the two would complement each other, like this recipe from the fifteenth-century Dutch text *Wel ende edelike spijse* (*Good and Noble Food*).

Greens (Dutch style)
Boil them and cut them (a selection of 'greens', like leeks, cabbage, kale, spinach etc.). Then grind pepper, sage, parsley and some bread crumbs, tempered [mixed] with the [boiling]water of the greens. Mix [together] in a pan and [add] a cup of wine.[25]

The following fifteenth-century English recipe, contains more herbs than anything else:

Whyte Wortes
Take of þe erbys lyke as þou dede for jouutes, and sethe hem in water tyl þey ben neyshe; þanne take hem vp, an bryse hem fayre on a bord, as drye as þow may; þan choppe hem smale, an caste hem on a potte, an ley hem with flowre of Rys; take mylke of almaundys, an cast þer-to, & hony, nowt to moche, þat it be nowt to swete, an safron & salt; an serue it forth ynne, ryȝth for a good potage.[26]

White herbs (my translation)
Take the herbs as you did for joutes (from the same manuscript this includes Borage, violets, marshmallow, parsley, young herbs, beets, avens (a member of the rose family), a type of hawk-weed and orach or mountain spinach). Boil them in water until soft. Take them out of the liquid and bruise and chop them finely on a board. Throw them into a pot with rice flour, almond milk and just enough honey to sweeten slightly. Add saffron and salt. Serve it forth as a good pottage.

There are numerous Islamic dishes with vegetables, like this one for *Jannâniyya*, which gardeners were alleged to have prepared directly in their flower or vegetable gardens. The following recipe is understood to have been written by the well-known poet and singer, Ibrahim ibn al-Mahdi, an Abbasid prince who was briefly proclaimed caliph of Baghdad in 817. It was published in *Kitab al-Tabeekh fi 'l-Maghrib wa 'l-Andalus fi 'Asr al-Muwahhidin* (*The Cookbook of al-Maghrib and Andalusia in the Era of the Almohads*). This is an anonymous thirteenth-century compilation written in Muslim Spain and translated into English in the 1980s.

Jannâniyya (the gardener's dish)

It was the custom among us to make this in the flower and vegetable gardens. If you make it in summer or fall, take saltwort, Swiss chard, gourd, small eggplants, 'eyes' of fennel, fox-grapes, the best parts of tender gourd and flesh of ribbed cucumber and smooth cucumber; chop all this very small, as vegetables are chopped, and cook with water and salt; then drain off the water. Take a clean pot and in it pour a little water and a lot of oil, pounded onion, garlic, pepper, coriander seed and caraway; put on a moderate fire and when it has boiled, put in the boiled vegetables. When it has finished cooking, add grated or pounded bread and dissolved [sour] dough, and break over it as many eggs as you are able, and squeeze in the juice of tender coriander and of mint, and leave on the hearthstone until the eggs set. If you make it in spring, then [use] lettuce, fennel, peeled fresh fava beans, spinach, Swiss chard, carrots, fresh cilantro and so on; cook it all and add the spices already indicated, plenty of oil, cheese, dissolved [sour] dough and eggs.

The next recipe appears in the fifteenth-century French manuscript *Le Recueil de Riom*. There is a category of herb in France termed 'fine herbs', so named for their delicate flavours, including chives, tarragon, chervil and parsley. 'English puree' sounds to me a bit like a fancy mushy pea dish that uses parsley and saffron for added flavour.[27]

La purée d'angleterre

Y fault lesser cuire les poiz tant qu'il soient bien cuis. Et mectre l'ongnon et le percilh monument mainssé avec et boullir ensemble, et du saffran, et du poivre, et du sel, et du vin aigre, du verjust.[28]

English puree
Leave peas to cook until they are well done. Take onions and parsley, cut into small pieces with it and boil together. Add saffron and pepper and salt and vinegar and verjuice.

Utilized in Chinese medicine, as an early form of painkiller and even for bee whispering, mushrooms, which grow wild in fields and forests have also been used extensively in cooking for thousands of years. Edible mushrooms were certainly eaten in ancient Egypt and even earlier among some South American civilizations. Roman leaders ensured their personal tasters prevented the consumption of any poisonous imposters, despite the fact that some species of fungi can take up to fourteen hours to manifest symptoms of poisoning.

Historically mushrooms have widely been regarded with suspicion. Druids and Vikings used them for their hallucinogenic properties. But it was during the two twentieth-century world wars that mushrooms gained their real reputation, as a plentiful source of accessible food throughout Europe.[29]

The recipe below dates to the 1600s, but 'funges' (fungi) were frequently enjoyed paired with other vegetables and herbs in Britain from early medieval times, despite the mushroom's murky reputation and confusion amongst some communities over its ability to materialize overnight!

Fricate champignons (fried mushrooms)

Make ready your champignons as you do for stewing, and when you have
poured away the black liquor that comes from them, put your champignons
into a Frying pan with a piece of sweet Butter, a little Parsley, Tyme, sweet Marjoram, a piece of Onion shred very small, a little Salt and fine beaten Pepper, so fry them till they be enough, so have ready the lear abovesaid, and put it to the champignons whilst they are in the Pan, toss them two or three times, put them forth and serve them.[30]

Before modern methods of canning and preserving, food was pickled, salted and cured. There has been a revival in recent years for fermented foods which heal the gut and repair the damage modern contemporary diets have precipitated. One of the most recognized of these foods is kimchi, an ancient Korean dish of fermented vegetables, of which there are numerous variations. The origins of kimchi – originally known as *chimchae*, extend at least 3,000 years and it has now become a national dish. There is even a museum located in Seoul dedicated to this seasoned fermented tradition, which is called Museum Kimchikan. Cabbage and radishes are the most popular ingredient, combined with salt, garlic, onions, ginger, chili peppers, carrots and other seasonings and oils, enriched with some type of seafood. It is only in the last few hundred years that spices have become integral to kimchi.

Eumsik Dimibang (*Understanding the Taste of Food*), written in Korea by Lady Jang Gye-hyang in the 1600s, is known to be one of the earliest cookbooks to be written by a woman in Asia and contains many recipes for fermented vegetables.

Good old piccalilli, based on Indian methods of pickling vegetables in spices, has also managed to stand the test of time, where many others have failed. This recipe for pickled cabbage appears in the 1616 edition of the Danish *Koge bog* (*Cookbook*)

To pickle cabbage
Chop it finely, sprinkle it well each layer by itself in a container or barrel. Between each layer sprinkle salt, cumin and juniper berries and put a good weight on it for 4 or 5 days. Thereafter pour vinegar over it.[31]

Glamorgan sausages are known today as a meat-free speciality; historically they contained pork and Glamorgan cheese, which evolved into Caerphilly, along with a variety of herbs and spices, making it a piquant sausage. In due course this sausage morphed into a vegetarian, skinless dish that could be prepared with any type of strong hard cheese, coated in breadcrumbs. The recipe included here is one from the twentieth century.

Glamorgan sausages

1 medium onion finely chopped
6 oz cheddar cheese
10 oz fresh breadcrumbs
Pinch of dried sage

Pinch of mustard powder
2 eggs separated.
Salt and pepper
Fresh breadcrumbs for coating
Oil for frying

Mix together the onion, cheese, breadcrumbs, sage, mustard, egg yolks, salt, and pepper. Divide the mixture into twelve pieces and roll each portion into a small sausage shape. Lightly beat the egg whites in a shallow bowl. Place the breadcrumbs on a large plate. Coat each sausage shape with egg white and then press on a coating of crumbs. Heat about an inch of oil in a large saucepan. Fry the sausages for five to seven minutes, or until golden brown, turning once. Drain on absorbent kitchen paper. Serve hot.[32]

Burdock root has been used in holistic medicine for centuries. It contains numerous antioxidants and has long been considered beneficial to the gut. Still eaten in Japan today, this recipe is sometimes referred to as 'cousins' on account of the fact that some of the ingredients are similar to each other.

Itoko-ni いとこに **(simmered cousins)**
Put in such things as *azuki* beans, *gobō* [sliced burdock root and carrot], *imo* [sweet potatoes], *daikon* [Japanese radish], *tofu* [roasted chestnuts] or *kuwai* [small Japanese tuber]. In *nakamiso* [a type of miso] is good. Since, in this way, you can simmer many various things, it is *itoko ni*.[33]

Pies, Tarts and Puddings

Pies, tarts and puddings make up some of the world's oldest staple dishes. With 'coffyns' of pastry once filled with all manner of sweet and savoury fillings and puddings referring to anything from boiled intestines to something like this sixteenth-century pudding made in a turnip root.

Pudding in a turnip root (transcribed by Mark and Jane Waks)
Take your Turnep root, and wash it fair in warm water, and scrape it faire and make it hollow as you doo a Carret roote, and make your stuffe of grated bread, and Apples chopt fine, then take Corance, and hard Egs,

and season it with Sugar Sinamon, and Ginger, and yolks of hard egs and so temper your stuffe, and put it into the Turnep, then take faire water, and set it on the fire, and let it boyle or ever you put in your Turneps, then put in a good peece of sweet Butter, and Claret Wine, and a little Vinagre, and Rosemarye, and whole Mace, Sugar, and Corance, and Dates quartered, and when they are boyled inough, then willl they be tender, then serve it in.[34]

Herb pie

Pick two handfuls of parsley from the stems, half the quantity of spinach, two lettuces, some mustard and cresses, a few leaves of borage and white beet-leaves; wash and boil them a little; then drain and press out of the water; cut them small; mix and lay them in a dish, sprinkle with some salt. Mix a batter of flour, two eggs well beaten, a pint of cream, and half a pint of milk, and pour it on the herbs, cover with a good crust and bake.[35]

Bistort was known to help a variety of ailments from diabetes to menstrual pains and infectious diseases. The leaves were gathered around March, dried and then pummelled down into a powder which were then mixed with a liquid.

Bistort or dock pudding is an old Cumbrian and Yorkshire dish, with the main ingredient being the leaves of bistort, sometimes known as gentle or passion dock. Traditionally eaten during Lent, this is a fried pudding, opposed to one baked or boiled. It became popular during the Second World War, but fried or boiled herb 'puddings' such as this have a legacy that extends right back to Roman times.

The World Dock Pudding contest takes place annually in the village of Mytholmroyd in West Yorkshire.

Passion dock pudding

Boil tender dock leave with green onions or spring onions (or if not available then ordinary onions). When cooked add a handful of oatmeal or wheatmeal, one beaten up egg and a teaspoon of butter or margarine. Simmer for half an hour.[36]

The subsequent recipe for French puffs is visually very striking. I have included a picture of this particular dish which I recreated using the original method.

To make French puffes with greene hearbes

Take Spinage, Parsley, Endife, a sprigge or two of Sauory: mince them very fine: season them with Nutmeg, Ginger, and Sugar. Wet them with Egges, according to the quantitie of the Hearbes, more or lesse. Then take the coare of a Lemmon, cut it in round slices very thinne: put to euery slice of your Lemmon one spoonefull of this stuffe. Then frye it with sweet Lard in a Frying panne as you frye Egges, and serue them with sippets or without, sprinckle them eyther with white Wine or Sacke, or any other Wine, sauing Rennish Wine.

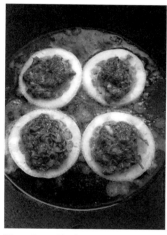

French puffs. (*Emma Kay*)

Serue them eyther at Dinner or Supper.[37]

If you want to make green pudding from 1658, I have modernized the recipe directly below the original, rechristening it boiled green dumplings.

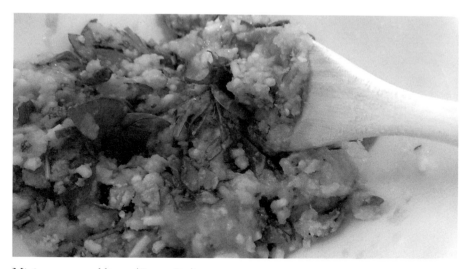

Mixing green puddings. (*Emma Kay*)

To make a green pudding

Take a penny loafe of stale Bread, grate it, put to halfe a pound of Sugar, grated Nutmeg, as much Salt as will season it, three quarters of a pound of beef-suet shred very small, then take sweet Herbs, the most of them Marigolds, eight Spinages: shred the Herbs very small, mix all well together, then take two Eggs and work them up together with your hand, and make them into round balls, and when the water boyles put them in, serve them with Rose-water, Sugar, and Butter or Sauce.[38]

Boiled green dumplings

80g breadcrumbs
50g sugar
60g shredded suet
A handful of spinach leaves (torn)
A handful of basil leaves (cut fine)
3 tsp tarragon (cut fine)
3 tsp thyme (cut fine)
Several sprigs of rosemary (cut fine)
A handful of parsley (chopped)
A pinch of nutmeg
A pinch of salt
2 eggs
Flour to coat

Mix together the breadcrumbs and sugar with the nutmeg and salt. Add the shredded suet, all the herbs and the spinach. Beat the eggs and use your hands to work them into the mixture (you can add a little plain flour at this stage if it is looking too moist). Make around 5 good meatball-sized rounds with the mixture and coat each one well with flour to create a crust.

Have a large pan of boiling water and a ladle. Lower the heat slightly. Gently lower each pudding into the water and hold in the ladle for a few seconds to maintain shape. Simmer for around 4/5 minutes. Take care to watch over them as they may start to break up after around 4/5 minutes.

Remove and serve with a sauce or a warming dish of choice.

Hortopitta (pie of greens), is a type of Greek Spanakopita, made with wild horta – generic leafy green herby vegetables, similar to, but more substantial than spinach or Swiss chard. Hortopitta would have been prepared in traditional round stone ovens or deep fried in olive oil.

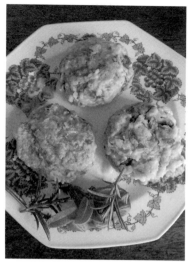

Green puddings. (*Emma Kay*)

In the Geek town of Methana, in a time-honoured way, women would come together to roll out the filo pastry and exchange gifts of hortas stored in the creases of their aprons.[39] Hortas are picked wild, as and when they are available and combined to include anything from dandelions to beetroot tops. A customary recipe for hortopitta will be similar to the one I have included here which was provided by an elder member of the community from the village of Loutses on Corfu.

To make a Hortopitta (horta pie) for 6 people

750g of various hortas
1 Tbsp each of fresh fennel leaves, dill weed and parsley
3 onions
100ml of oil
250g of feta cheese
3 eggs
100ml of milk
2 Tbsp of uncooked rice
Salt and pepper
8 sheets or 200g of filo pastry

Boil 3 litres of water in a very large saucepan with 2 tablespoons of salt. When the water is bubbling fiercely, put in the spinach and horta and let it boil for two or three minutes. Drain it for fifteen minutes and then chop it finely. Chop the fennel leaves, dill weed, parsley and onions finely and fry them gently in half the oil until the onions yellow. Add them to the chopped greens with the rice and all but two tablespoons of the milk. Beat two of the eggs with the white of the third egg and add them to the vegetables. Mix everything together thoroughly.

Take a rectangular baking tray, sized about 28cm by 35cm, with sides at least 8cm deep, and moisten it with oil. Lie a leaf of filo over the bottom of the tray and brush it with oil. Grate or chop the feta very finely and divide into eight piles. Scatter one pile of feta over the filo. Lay three more leaves of filo pastry on top, brushing each one with oil and sprinkling each with cheese, then smooth the vegetable mixture on top of everything. If the filo leaves are larger than the pan, oil the side of each overlapping leaf and fold them over the horta, sprinkling on more cheese. Lay a new leaf of filo over everything, brush it with oil, sprinkle it with cheese and repeat the procedure twice more. Lay on the last filo leaf and brush it with a mixture of the remaining milk and the last egg yolk. Score the top few layers of the filo with a sharp knife, making four parallel incisions from side to side of the tray. Bake it in a moderate oven for 40 minutes or until the pastry is golden. Let it cool for 5 minutes before cutting into rectangular slices.[40]

Written around 1350, *Daz buch von guter spise*, or *The Book of Good Eating*, is understood to represent the oldest example of a German cookbook. Written for and by the wealthy, urban and cosmopolitan spheres of German society, it provides tremendous insight into early medieval European cuisine, which was, as we know, infused with a variety of herbs. It is also a book containing several mock or parody recipes, which apparently was a genuine aspect of some medieval medical and dietetic texts.

Take the following recipe which is taken directly from *Daz buch von guter spise* and written in rhyming couplets:

Ein guot gerihte, der ez gern izzel
Will du machen ein guot bigeriht,
So nim sydeln sweyz,
Daz macht den magen gar heiz,
Und nim kiseiinges smaltz,
Daz ist den meidenguot, die do sin hueffehaltz.
Und nim bromber und bresteling,
Daz ist daz aller beste ding.

Bist du niht an sinnen taup,
So nim gruen wingart laup.
du soit nemen binzen,
lubstickel und minzen,
daz sint guote würtze
füer die grozzen fürtze.
nim stigelitzes versen, und mucken füozze,
daz macht daz köestlin allez süezze,
daz ist guot und mag wol sin
ein guot lecker spigerihtelin.
Ach und versaltz nur niht,
wanne ez ist ein guot geriht.

A good dish that you will like
If you want to prepare a good side dish,
Take pints of sweat,
This makes the stomach quite hot,
And take pebble grease,
This is good for maidens who are lame in the hips.
And take blackberries and strawberries,
This is the best tiling.
If you are not deaf on your senses
Take green vine-leaves.
You should take rush,
Lovage and mint.
These are good seasonings
For the big farts.
Take goldfinch-heels and flies' feet,
This makes the little dish very sweet,
This is good and may well be
A tasty little vomiting-dish.
Oh, and just don't add too much salt,
Since it is a good dish.[41]

I marvel at the satire of this addition to the book, which very blatantly
pokes fun at medieval culinary literature, reminding us that some of the
concoctions and paired ingredients of the time, were in fact often bizarre

and slightly ridiculous. I find it reassuring somehow that there was an awareness of the pretention of early recipe writing, the advice of which, was clearly not always taken literally.

Also from Germany, *Das Kuchbuch der Sabina Welserin* (*Sabina Welsarin's Cookbook*) written in the 1500s, contains a lovely, simple recipe for herb tart.

Ain kraúttorten

> *Zúm ersten nim jspen ain hendlin voll, deýmenten, mangoldt, salúa, das mangoldt soll 3 mal mer sein als der anderen kreúter/ nach dem man die torten grosß will haben, nim púterschmaltz, rest die vorgemelten kreúter woll darin, nim ziwiben, klaine weinberlen, zúcker, als vil dich gút donckt, nim acht air, klopffs woll jn das obgemelt vorgeschriben vnd mach ain boden mit ainem aý vnd bachs langsam.*[42]

Herb tart (translation by David Friedman)
First of all, take one handful of sage, a handful of marjoram and some lavender and rosemary, also a handful of chard, and chop it together; take six eggs, sugar, cinnamon, cloves, raisins and rose water and let it bake.[43]

In contrast to the modest little tart above, I discovered the recipe below in the French manuscript of 1420, *Du fait de cuisine* by Master Chiquart Amiczo, chef to Amadeus VIII, Duke of Savoy, also known as Pope Felix V. It is an elaborate and extravagant example of a typical medieval meat, fruit, herb and spice concoction gorged by wealthy noblemen. The book offers detailed descriptions of how to prepare and organize feasts, while outlining the specifics of one feast in particular, given in honour of Mary of Burgundy, the wife of Amadeus III. The original manuscript is held in the archives of Valais, Switzerland. It has been digitized and translated only a couple of times. I am including this recipe as it is rarely reproduced, provides a prime example of European medieval repasts and contains at least four types of herbs, including hyssop, which was more often to be found in soups or stews. I do not know whether these tarts were originally from Parma in Italy and I can find no other recipes for this type of tart, although it resembles the medieval Chewettes, a dish of finely chopped meats or fish, which were mixed with spices, herbs and fruit before being baked. Of course, Parma tarts may be a descendant of the Italian torta parmigiana, or a parmesan pie, particularly as this recipe contains cheese.

Parma tarts

For the said parma tarts which are ordered to be made, to give you understanding, take three or four large pigs and, if the feast should be larger than I think, let one take more, and from these pigs remove the heads and the hams, and put the fat apart to be melted; and take the said pigs and cut them into fair slices or pieces and wash them very well and put them to cook in fair and clean cauldrons, and put in salt in measure. And for the said parma tarts you will need three hundred pigeons, two hundred very young chickens – and if it happens that the feast is given at a time when there are no very young chickens, have one hundred young capons – six hundred small birds; and these pigeons, poultry, and small birds should be plucked and cleaned properly and cleanly; and take the pigeons and split them in half, and also split the poultry and cut it in quarters; and then take the pigeons, poultry, and small birds and put into fair small casks, wash properly and cleanly three or four times in fair and clean water, and then put them to boil in fair and clean cauldrons, and put in salt in measure; and check that it does not cook too much; and, being cooked subtly, draw out your meat into fair and clean *cornues* [dishes made from horns] and put your small birds in one place and the other meat in another. And then take your pork fat and cut a great deal of it and put into fair and clean pans and melt well and, being well melted, strain it into other fair and clean pans; and then take your small birds and sauté them in your lard lightly and not too much, and also next the other meat. And of figs six pounds and six pounds of dates, of pine nuts six pounds, of prunes six pounds, of raisins eight pounds; and then take your figs, prunes, and dates and cut them fine – as small as the smallest raisins – and remove the stems from the raisins and clean them well. And then take your pine nuts and rub them very well, then winnow them on fair platters; then put them on a fair cloth and pick them over and clean them well and properly so that there remains nothing but the white nutmeat. And then put your figs, prunes, raisins, dates, and pine nuts into a fair, white and clean *cornue*, and let it be well covered with a fair, white and clean cloth so that nothing which is not clean falls therein. And then arrange that you have herbs, that is sage, parsley, hyssop, and marjoram, of which have such a large amount of parsley that you have a great bowl full drained and with the leaves stripped off the stems, and sage, hyssop, and marjoram added in measure; then put them in a fair and clean *cornue*, and wash them well and properly in three or four changes of fresh water, and then put them on fair and clean boards and chop them very small. And check to see if your pork is cooked and put it on fair tables, and you should have your fair, large and very flat boards; and you who are making this fair parma tart, together with the assistants which you have assigned to it, take care to remove the skin of the said pigs and let no bones remain, and chop your meat very small; and in chopping your said meat take herbs and put them in with your meat; and then have a large, fair, clean and clear *bacine* [basin] and put your said meat therein – and to give understanding of what the basin is, I mean that this should be a fair and large pan of those in which one cooks big and large fish. And then arrange that you have a quintal of best Crampone or Brie cheese or the best cheese which can be found, and then take the said cheese and pare and clean it well and properly, and cut it small, then bray it in a mortar very well and strongly; then take six hundred eggs and moisten your cheese therewith in braying, and continually sprinkle with the said eggs so that they are well bound and moistened and according to the quantity of the parma tarts which you are ordered to make. And take the pan which I described to you above, and put therein lard which is refined in which one has sautéed the meat, and put it in according to the quantity of the stuff which you have, and let it be put over a fair clear fire; and have two good strong assistants stirring the filling strongly and firmly with a great slotted spoon with two hands, and then let it down over a fair fire of clear coals; and let your figs, prunes, dates, raisins, pine nuts, cut as is said above, be washed two or three times in fair, clean and clear water and then afterward washed in good white wine and then put to drain and dry on fair and clean boards; and then, being drained, throw it into your filling, and let it be very well stirred in; and then take your cheese which has been brayed and moistened with egg as is said above – the quantity which you have made for the said filling – and put into your filling while braying well and strongly; and take the said pan off the fire. And take your spices, white ginger, fine powder, grains of paradise, saffron to give colour, and put in cloves in measure, put them therein and stir continually; and have a great deal of sugar beaten into powder and throw in a great deal according to the quantity of the filling, and stir continually. And arrange that you have fair and clean pans, or if you find fair and clean ceramic dishes take as many as you need to make your parma tarts in such great quantity that you will have some left over; and then when you have your fair and clean pans or ceramic dishes arrange that you have two or three thousand sugared wafers, and then take your pans or your ceramic dishes and take some of the lard in which you fried your small birds and poultry and put into your pans or ceramic dishes and then take your wafers and put in each dish on the bottom and around it a layer of the said wafers so that there are four or five one on another; and on the said wafers take of the said filling and make a layer, and then on top of the filling put the small birds here and there and not together; and put between two small birds a quarter of a pigeon and elsewhere a quarter chicken between two small birds, and do this in such manner that of small birds, quarter pigeons and quarter chickens there is made well and adroitly a layer set on top of the layer of the filling; and on top of this layer made of small birds, quarter pigeons, and quarter chickens is made another layer of the said filling, and on top of this layer made of filling put wafers in the fashion and manner which is said above as they were put on the bottom of the said pan or ceramic dish; and, this being done, they should be covered well and properly with the said wafers. Then take cold lard and put on top, and then put your tarts in the oven which has been well heated; and you will be well advised when they cook to have leaves of spinach and white chard well cleaned and washed so that, if the said wafers burn at all, you can put them on top. And then draw out your parma tarts and scrape them well and properly so that there remains nothing burned, and then put them on fair serving dishes; and, with them on the serving dishes, take your gold leaf and put it on your parma tarts in the manner of a chessboard, and powdered sugar on top. And when one serves it, let on each tart be put a little banner with the arms of each lord who is served these parma tarts.[44]

The following recipe for angelica apple pie from the 1930s is originally from Lancashire. Despite largely associating this vivid green herb as the candied variety frequently added to florentines, angelica also complements both apple and rhubarb very well.

Angelica apple pie

For the biscuit crust:
8 oz self-raising flour
5 oz margarine
1 tsp of caster sugar
1 egg yolk
Some water with squeezed lemon juice.

Sift the flour and sugar together and rub in the margarine. Add the lemon water a bit at a time until you get a dry paste. Turn onto a floured board and roll out.

For the filling:
4 large cooking apples
4 oz angelica (stalks of)
4 Tbsp caster sugar
The juice of half a lemon
½ tsp of grated nutmeg

Peel and grate the apples and cut the peeled angelica into small pieces. Add the sugar, lemon juice and nutmeg. Roll out the biscuit crust and line a pie plate with it. Put in the fruit filling and bake in a moderate oven (180°C/356°F) for 30 minutes. Serve with whipped cream.[45]

Fish Dishes

All the ingredients in this category are commonly associated with the ancient eating rituals of Lent and constitute a large percentage of many a medieval cookbook.

Eels are cited as a staple food in Britain, as far back as the Domesday Book. In the later Middle Ages they were typically seasoned and baked in salt and pepper, with shallots , sage and marjoram and added to pies and pottages. The English professional chef Robert May included numerous recipes in his cookbook of the Restoration era, *The Accomplisht Cook*.

Several hundred years later, eels were as popular as ever and frequently coupled with a variety of herbs, like this recipe for eel soup in William Kitchener's acclaimed *Cook's Oracle*.

Eel soup

Take a couple of middling-sized onions, cut them in half, and cross your knife over them two or three times; put two ounces of butter into a stew-pan; when it is melted, put in the onions, stir them about until they are lightly browned – cut into pieces three pounds of unskinned eels, put them into your stew pan, and shake them over the fire for five minutes; then add three quarters of boiling water, and when they come to a boil, take the scum off very clean, then put in a quarter of an ounce of the green leaves (not dried) of winter savoury, the same of lemon thyme, and twice the quantity of parsly, two drachms of allspice, the same of black pepper – cover it close, and let it boil gently for two hours, then strain it off, and skim it very clean. To thicken it, put three ounces of butter into a clean stew-pan; when it is melted, stir in as much flour as will make it a stiff paste, then add the liquor by degrees, let it simmer for ten minutes and pass it through a sieve, then put your soup on in a clean stew-pan – and have ready some little square pieces of fish fried of a nice light brown – either eels, soles, plaice or skate will do; the fried fish should be added about ten minutes before the soup is served up. Forcemeat balls are sometimes added.[46]

Written in the tenth century by Abu Muhammad al-Muthaffar ibn Nasr ibn Sayyār al-Warrāq, *Kitab al-tabikh* (*Book of Dishes*) is understood to be the oldest surviving Arabic cookbook. It has been translated several times into different languages. Known for the culinary spice and herb fusions, it was undoubtedly Eastern methods of healing that greatly influenced the advancement of European medicine. Whether the subsequent recipe for jaundice proved to be an effective remedy is contentious:

Fish recipe for jaundice

Take *ukshuth* (twining, leafless plants), the pulp of a small and smooth cucumber, sprigs of rue, a small amount of parsley and fresh leeks. Chop them all into fine pieces. Stuff the cavity of a fish with this mixture and bake it or cook it in vinegar or any other liquid. It is a tried-and-true cure. God willing.[47]

Stewed trout

Take a large Trout fair trimm'd, and wash it, and put it into a deep pewter dish, then take half a pint of sweet Wine, with a lump of butter, & a little whole Mace, Parsley, Savory, & Thyme, mince them all small, and put them into the Trouts belly, and so let it stew a quarter of an hour, then mince the yelk of a hard Egg, and strew it on the Trout, and laying the herbs about it, and scraping on Sugar, serve it up.[48]

Sansho is a type of Japanese pepper, used historically for both medicinal and culinary purposes. Typically used to treat diarrhoea and other digestive issues it is also used in cooking in a similar way to that of Chinese Sichuan pepper.

Ryōri Monogatari was published in 1643 by an unnamed author. It is understood to be one of Japan's oldest published cookbooks. The following recipe for roasted salmon with whole sansho seeds, or Sake no iriyaki 鮭 のいりやき, is taken from *Ryōri Monogatari*:

Sake no iriyaki
Make as you would for *sugiyaki* (which is another recipe featured in the book):

Sugiyaki
Cut *tai* [sea bream] thick and put it aside. Darken *miso* in *dashi* [a type of Japanese stock] and add to a pot. When it is simmering put it in the box [made from cedar wood]. To start with, add the bones and head and simmer. Put the body meat in only briefly. Pour in *dobu*. [fried liver and vegetables]. Prepare and put in oysters, *hamaguri* [clams], *tōfu*, [Tofu], *nebuka*, or other things outside those.

Sake no iriyaki (continued)
Grind up half of the [fish] eggs and put it aside. Put aside the other half as they are. Season with *dashi-tamari* [a basic Japanese broth], put in the intestines and liver with the meat and simmer. When it is about a standing boil, put in the ground and whole eggs. Arrange, and then serve shortly. It is good to add whole *sanshō* seeds.[49]

Issac (Izaak) Walton's carp
Izaack Walton was an English writer of the seventeenth century, best known for his book *The Compleat Angler*. The following recipe is taken from this publication, detailing how best to cook carp:

Take Carp (alive if possible); scour him, and rub him clean with water and salt, but scale him not; then open him; and put him, with his blood and his liver, which you must save when you open him, into a small pot or kettle: then take sweet marjoram, thyme and parsley, of each half a handful; a sprig of rosemary, and another of savory; bind them into two or three mall bundles, and put them to your carp, with four or five whole onions, twenty pickled oysters, and three anchovies. Then pour upon your carp as much claret wine as will only cover him: and season your claret well with salt, cloves, and mace and the rinds of oranges and lemons. That done, cover your pot and set it on a quick fire, till it be sufficiently boiled. Then take out the carp; and lay it, with the broth, into the dish; and pour upon it a quarter of a pound of the best fresh butter, melted and beaten with half a dozen spoonfuls of the broth, the yolks of two or three eggs, and some of the herbs shred: garnish your dish with lemons, and so serve it up.[50]

Egg Dishes

Erbolates [1]. XX. VIII. XII

Take parsel, myntes [2], sauerey, & sauge, tansey, veruayn, clarry, rewe, ditayn, fenel, southrenwode, hewe hem & grinde hem smale, medle hem up with Ayrenn. do butter in a trape. & do þe fars þerto. & bake it & messe it forth.[51]

Herbolade or a confection of herbs (my translation)

Take parsley, mint, savory and sage, tansy, vervain, clary, rue, dittany, fennel and southernwood. Chop them and grind them small. Mix them up with eggs, butter a pie pan and add the mix to the pan. Season, bake and serve.

The following recipe is taken from a fifteenth-century collection of recipes from Southern Italy. The cult of the Virgin Mary has dominated the lives of many communities for centuries and there are numerous herbs associated with her, so it is difficult to determine the specifics here for translation purposes. Rosemary is so called from the 'rose of Mary' and there is one legend that tells of the Virgin Mary fleeing the holy land and throwing her robes on a bush of rosemary in Egypt, which turned the flowers from white to blue and led to the herb becoming associated with its abilities to challenge evil. Rosemary was also worn by couples at weddings in ancient Greece and Rome.

Herb fritters

Bone sondo le frictelle de pane grassuto con herbe sancte Marie overo menta et petrosimuli assai. Stemperali colle ova assay et con uno poco de aqua et falle frigere con uno poco de lardo. Sendò se tennesse bene, micti uno poco de farina.

Good are the fritters of bread immersed in grease (oil or butter) with the herb holy Mary or else mint and stone parsley enough. Temper them with enough eggs and with a little water and fry them with a little lard. In order that they hold well, put a little flour.[52]

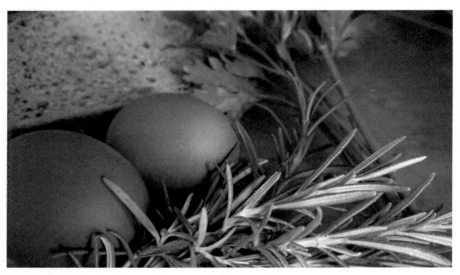

Ingredients for herb fritters with rosemary. (*Emma Kay*)

Tansy is a herb long associated with birth and as such was often made into cakes at Easter; its other link to this time of year is tansy's alleged abilities to counteract heavy phlegm and parasitic worms, both arising from the over-consumption of seafood throughout the period of Lent. Cakes made with tansy were popular for several centuries. This one from the 1500s is a typical example:

Tansy cake

> Breke egges in bassyn, and swynge hem sone,
> Do powder of peper therto anone,
> Then grynde *tansay*, tho juse owte wrynge,

To blynde with tho egges, withowte lesynge.
In pan or skelet thou shalt hit frye,
In buttur well skymm et wyturly,
Or white grece thou may take therto,
Geder hit on acake, thenne hase thou do,
With platere of tre, and frye hit browne,
On brodeleches serve hit thou schalle,
With fraunche-mele [eggs and sheep's fat] or other metis withalle.[53]

Published in 1520, the Spanish *Libre del Coch* or the *Book of Cooking*, was written in Catalan by a cook to the king of Naples, who may or may not have been Ruperto de Nola. It was republished numerous times and was very popular. The following recipes for eggs appeared in the 1529 edition. Much Spanish cooking benefitted from the wisdom of the Arabs during this time.

Potaje de alideme de huevos (egg alideme stew)

Take a casserole that is very clean, and cast into it onions, and parsley, and mint, and marjoram, which is called *moraduj* in the kingdoms of Aragon, with salt and oil, all mixed with water, and set it all to cook; and when it is cooked, grind a little of these herbs, that have cooked in the pot or casserole, with a little of that same onion. And when they are ground, blend them with the same broth; and when they are blended, set them to cook in a clean pot. And then take egg yolks, and beat them very well with verjuice or white vinegar; and cast into the pot all fine spices, and ground saffron, more rather than less; and when it has cooked a little, remove it from the fire. And leave it a little while to rest or cool; and then cast in the eggs little by little; then return it to the fire; and when it has cooked a little while longer, remove it from the fire and stir it well constantly and in such a manner that never ceases while it boils.[54]

Torta de huevos que se dice salivate (egg cake said to salivate)

Take some sage leaves, and grind them quite vigorously; and take a good quantity of eggs, and beat them and mix them with the sage; and then take a frying pan, and cast in lard in such a manner that after melting there is a finger's breadth or more in the frying pan; and if there is no lard, take common oil which is sweet and very good, the same quantity;

and when the lard or oil boils, cast in the eggs with the sage, and make of them an omelet which is well cooked; and this omelet should be two fingers thick, or more. And when it is well cooked or fried, cast it on a good plate with much sugar above and below; and this omelet should be eaten hot.[55]

While not strictly a cookbook, *Le Ménagier de Paris* (*The Householder of Paris*) was a guidebook for women, especially wives, outlining their duties during the early medieval period. Written in 1393, the book contains all manner of information from how to take care of the household to what to cook.

Divers (various) ways of preparing eggs

One herbolace (arboulastre) or two of eggs. Take of dittany two leaves only, and of rue less than the half of naught, for know that it is strong and bitter; of smallage, tansey, mint and sage, of each some four leaves or less, for each is strong; marjoram a little more, fennel more, parsley more still; but of porray, beets, violet leaves, spinach, lettuces, and clary, as much of the one as of the others, until you have two large handfuls. Pick them over and wash them in cold water, then dry them of all the water, and bray two heads of ginger; then put your herbs into the mortar two or three times and bray them with the ginger. And then have sixteen eggs well beaten together, yolks and whites, and bray and mix them in the mortar with the things abovesaid, then divide it into two, and make two thick omelettes, which you shall fry as followeth. First you shall heat your frying pan very well with oil, butter, or such other fat as you will, and when it is very hot all over all over and especially towards the handle, mingle and spread your eggs over the pan and turn them often over and over with a flat palette, then cast good grated cheese on the top; and know that it is so done, because if you grate cheese with the herbs and the eggs, when you come to fry your omlette, the cheese at the bottom will stick to the pan; and thus it befalls with an egg omlette if you mix the eggs with the cheese. Wherefor you should first put the eggs in the pan, and put the cheese on the top and then cover the edges with eggs; and otherwise it will cling to the pan. And when your herbs be cooked in the pan, cut your herbolace into a round or a square and eat it not too hot nor too cold.[56]

Meat Dishes

Interestingly, thyme was traditionally added to dishes to make them taste less fatty, which is why it features in so many Mediterranean meat dishes. Once the principal food of the wealthy, meat was typically flavoured with herbs to mask the taste of decomposition pre-refrigeration; they were less prestigious than spices which were habitually added to meat to denote wealth and status and game was the fare of nobility.

It is the Scandinavians who yielded the earliest known European cookbook, *Libellus de arte coquinaria* (*The Little Book of Culinary Arts*). It has been translated at least twice, by Henning Larson in the 1930s and again in the early twenty-first century by Rudolph Grewe and Constance Hieatt. Written by royal physician Henrik Haerpestaeng, the book is a compilation of four different versions containing recipes written in Danish, German and Icelandic and it forms part of a much broader manuscript of seven parts including sections on charms, sea depths, a book of herbal remedies, a book of antidotes, a book on gemstones and the cookbook. It is understood that some of the recipes have a legacy that extends to the twelfth century. As to be expected, the manuscript is full of quirky medieval beliefs. A method to determine whether or not a sick man would die, involved rubbing his feet with pork, which was then fed to the dog. If the dog ate the pork, the man would live, if the dog rejected the meat the man would surely die.[57]

The recipe below has been extracted from *Libellus de arte coquinaria*:

Chicken Pasty – Recipe XXX [W66]

Next, one should cut another hen in two. Make two sheets of dough out of flour and water. Put chopped bacon on them [the chicken pieces] and add whole sage leaves, and pepper and salt to taste. Wrap it in the pastry sheets and bake it as a roast. These are hen pasties.[58]

My version

Hot water crust pastry made with:
110g of lard
280g of water
500g of plain flour
2 tsp salt

Melt the lard in the water while slowly bringing to the boil. Sieve the flour and salt and add the hot lard and water mix. Mix until you form a stiff dough and leave to rest for a few minutes.

2 large chicken breasts filleted
About 100g of chopped pancetta
Large fresh sage leaves
Salt and pepper

Roll out the pastry into two sheets large enough for each chicken breast. Spread the pancetta and sage onto both sheets of pastry and season with salt and pepper. Place each chicken breast onto the centre of each sheet of pastry. Season again with salt and pepper. Fold the pastry over each chicken breast making sure to seal both ends, like an envelope. Place each parcel on a baking tray lined with baking paper and prick the tops of each one. Bake for around 40 minutes to 1 hour at 190°C/375°F.

One of the oldest surviving Polish cookbooks is Stanislaw Czerniecki's *Compendium Ferculorum albo zebranie potraw* (*Collection of Dishes*), published in 1682 in Krakow. Czerniecki was head chef to a noble family, the Lubomirskas. Having failed to find a copy in English, I was able to determine from my own poor translation skills that many recipes contained herbs, from cold fish in parsley and dill, using oil, pepper and cream, to a spinach cake again using dill and rosemary in Polish chicken soup. According to Robert and Maria Strybel, marjoram is Poland's most widely used seasoning, second only to pepper.[59] An established Polish dish was recorded in his book, *Ein new Kochbuch* (*A New Cookbook*) much earlier, in the 1500s, by chef, Marx Rumpolt, who had spent time cooking in Poland. The loin or saddle of

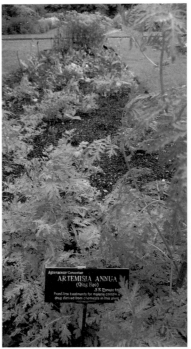

Chinese medicinal herb Qing hao at Oxford Botanic Garden and Arboretum. (*Emma Kay*)

veal was scored, marinated overnight in spring water, wine vinegar, garlic and marjoram. The meat was then seared on a spit, before being pot-roasted with kidneys in butter and more of the marinade. It was finally served in a pepper sauce.[60]

Chinese culinary practices represent some of the earliest and most documented in this genre, with origins as far back as the third century BC, with each era having its own progressive ideas. A fourteenth-century court nutritionist called Hu Sihui wrote *Yinshan Zhengyao* (*Principles for Drinking and Feasting*), a manual for the Chinese Mongol Empire. Great emphasis was placed on not mixing certain foods, such as rabbit and ginger, a combination which was thought to encourage cholera.

Astragalus membranaceus (*Huangqi*) is a herb which has been used in traditional Chinese medicine for thousands of years, to cure a variety of disorders. The following recipe has been taken from *Suiyuan Shidan* (*The Way of Eating*), a gastronomic manual written by the poet and scholar Yuan Mei sometime in the 1700s. The text was very recently translated into English for the first time by Sean J. S. Chen and the following recipe for chicken steamed with Huangqi, was thought to cure tuberculosis. Note that a 'liang' is an old Chinese unit of weight, equivalent to about 38g, or 50g in modern-day China.

Chicken steamed with Huangqi for curing tuberculosis

Take a chicken that is still too young to lay eggs and slaughter it. Do not rinse it with water. Remove the chicken's innards and stuff its cavity with one liang of Huangqi. Place the chicken on a wok with a rack made of chopsticks to steam. Cover the wok and seal it well. When the chicken is done, remove it from the wok. The collected juice from the chicken is unctuous and savoury, and can be used to treat weakness and fatigue resulting from the disease.[61]

Chicken and pork were the most commonly eaten meats of the past and this recipe for pigs in sauce, must have been piglets, considering that more than one is required for the dish.

Pygges in sawse

Take Pigges yskaldid and quarter hem and seeþ hem in water and salt, take hem and lat hem kele. take persel sawge. and grynde it with brede and zolkes of ayrenn harde ysode. temper it up with vyneger sum what thyk. and, lay the Pygges in a vessell. and the sewe onoward and serue it forth.

Pigs in sauce (my translation)
Take scalded pigs and quarter them and boil them in salted water; take them out and let them cool; take parsley, sage and grind it with bread and hard-boiled egg yolks, mix it up with vinegar to make it thick, and put the pigs in a vessel and pour the broth over the surface of the pigs and serve it.[62]

Portuguese method of dressing a loin of pork
Steep it during an entire week in red wine (claret in preference) with a strong infusion of garlic and a little spice; then sprinkle it with fine herbs, envelope it in bay leaves and bake it along with Seville oranges *piques de girofle* [clove-encrusted].[63]

Borage for a Transylvanian prince
If your prince or lord is sick, boil some borage like this. Wash the borage, clean it in warm water, then squeeze out the water, cook some beef or lamb in a small pipkin. Once the meat is half cooked, put the borage into it with some mace, add some vinegar and a bit of black pepper. Ask the doctor, for it is no shame to learn new things.[64]

The following recipe is taken from the tenth-century Islamic *Kitab al-Ṭabīḫ*, by Sayyar al-Warraq. It is both a culinary and medicinal dish to aid phlegmatic diarrhoea:

Masus (meat cooked in vinegar)
Boil chicken, qanabir [larks] and asafir [sparrows]. Stuff their cavities with a mix of parsley, rue and na'na' [a type of mint]; as well as seeds of anise, caraway, cumin and coriander, all fried. Add to these nankhawah [ajowan spice] and thyme. Boil the birds [again] in vinegar that has been left overnight to steep in thyme, cumin, cassia and black pepper then strained. It is good and very effective, God willing.[65]

The South African medicinal herb buchu is used in the food industry to enhance the flavour of blackcurrant. It is also famed for its antiseptic and inflammatory abilities. Due to its slightly minty flavour, buchu is often traditionally paired with lamb. 'Lamb and Mutton South Africa' is a South African organization responsible for educating consumers about these particular meats. The following recipe for rooibos- and buchu-infused lamb shanks is taken from their website.

Rooibos and buchu-infused lamb shanks served with creamy amasi samp

Yield: 4 portions
Preparation time: 45 minutes
Cooking time: 6 hours

INGREDIENTS:
4 lamb shanks
Salt, for seasoning
Large drizzle olive oil
1 onion
1 handful fresh thyme, chopped
3 garlic cloves, crushed/whole
2 Tbsp tomato paste
2 tsp ground pepper
3 cups beef/vegetable stock
1 cup red wine (dry)
2 tspn sugar
1 Tbspn rooibos tea leaves
1 tspn buchu tea leaves
2 bay leaves

For the creamy samp:
600ml samp
500ml water, for rinsing samp
2 potatoes
2 Tbsp original Aromat
3 cups chicken/vegetable stock/water
½ cup fresh cream
2 Tbsp amasi
Butter

METHOD (Lamb):

1. Preheat the oven to 140°C.
2. Season the lamb shanks with salt then fry in a little olive oil in a heavy-based saucepan, until brown on all sides. Work in batches so the pan isn't crowded. Remove and set aside.
3. Add a little more oil to the saucepan and sauté the onions and thyme for about 10 minutes until soft. Add the garlic, tomato paste and pepper and cook for another 2 to 3 minutes. Add the wine, tea leaves, sugar, stock and bring to a simmer.
4. Pour sauce over the lamb shanks in the roasting pan and cover tightly with a lid or with foil. The liquid should come about halfway up the shanks. Top with more water/stock if sauce is not enough.
5. Braise in the oven for 2 hours, or until the meat falls easily from the bone.
6. Remove the lamb from the sauce and remove as much fat from the sauce as you can. Discard the bay leaves and place sauce in a pot onto stove.
7. Simmer sauce over medium heat until thickened to your desired consistency.
8. Serve the lamb shanks topped with the sauce and creamy amasi samp.

METHOD (Samp):

1. Rinse samp and discard water.
2. In a slow cooker, put samp, potatoes, Aromat and stock and leave it to cook until soft and the water/stock has completely evaporated, about 6 hours.
3. Mix samp, fresh cream and amasi and stir well. Before serving, stir in butter.[66]

The *Florentine Codex* is a research project that was conducted by a Franciscan friar, Bernardino de Sahagu, documenting the communities of Mexico in the 1500s. The manuscript was so named, as it was initially housed in the city of Florence following its completion. References to both herbal remedies and the preparation of food can be found in this medieval Aztec anthology. One such recipe combines the two, as a remedy for the contraction of the knees:

When the knees start to contract, anoint them with the juice of the plants xiuhtontli or tzitzicton, yamanqui te-xochitl which should be crushed down in hawk's blood and that of a bird called the huacton. Place the patient in a bath while they eat the cooked feet of the hawk, the huachtli, a rabbit and a hare. After that boil a cockerel, also to be eaten, while some of the bird is mashed up with goose grease. Also to be consumed. The patient then needs to abstain from sex, avoid sleep and not over-eat.[67]

In some Portuguese-speaking countries including Brazil, chopped parsley and chopped spring onions together make an essential herb dish called *cheiro-verde*. It is sold everywhere in bundles as a readymade mix. The following recipe is taken from *Um tratado da cozinha portuguesa do século XV* or *A Treatise of Portuguese Cuisine from the 15th Century*. The predominant herbs used in wealthier Portuguese kitchens during the Middle Ages included coriander, parsley and mint, which were complemented with citrus juices, vinegars, onions and pine nuts.[68]

Picadinho de carne de vaca
Lavem carne devaca bem macia, e piquem-na bem miudinha. A seguir adicionem-lhe cravo, açafrão, pimenta, gengibre, cheiro-verde bem cortadinho, cebola batida, vinagre e sal. Refoguem tudo no azeite, e deixem cozinhar até secar a água. Sirvam sobre fatias de pão.

Beef mince
Wash the tender cow's meat, and mince it well. Next add cloves, saffron, blackpepper, ginger, well-chopped cheiro-verde [parsley], crushed onion, vinegar and salt. Sautee everything in the olive oil, and let cook until it the juices dry. Serve over sliced bread.[69]

Written in 1500 by Giyath Shah, ruler of Malwa, *Ninnatnama*, or the *Book of Delights*, includes a range of medieval Indian recipes, including the following for mutton:

Take the sheep complete with bones and wash it well and having added asafoetida (giant fennel), onions, fresh ginger, salt, fresh greens and fresh coriander, cook it. Put in plenty of water. Add some pepper and lime juice and when it is well cooked, take it off and either eat it as it is, or else flavour with more asafoetida essence.[70]

Crubeens, a derivative of the Irish word for hoof – *crúisc* – were once standard pub and street food fare in Ireland, typically served with stout and soda bread. This recipe for crubeens and boxty (pig's feet and potato dumplings) is from 1911, probably around the time that the dish began to go out of fashion, although it has made a bit of a revival in restaurants across Ireland in the last few years.

Crubeens and boxty

Boil three pickled pig's feet with a sliced carrot, half a sliced turnip, a sliced onion, a few fine herbs and a little white pepper and salt. When quite tender take out the long bones, and cut the meat into neat fillets about two inches long by one broad.

Make some forcemeat by mincing three quarters of a pound very lean pork, half a pound of fat bacon, four young green onions or shallots, and a little parsley, and season with a small saltspoonful of pepper, same quantity of grated nutmeg, and a good quarter of an ounce of salt. Pound altogether very smoothly, then work in a couple of eggs.

Cover the fillets with a thin coating of this mixture, and wrap up each neatly in a piece of pig's caul; grill over or in front of a moderate fire for about half an hour, being careful not to scorch the fillets. Serve with boxty, a shallot and parsley sauce in a sauce-boat, and parboiled potatoes cut in thin slices and fried in dripping.[71]

Sweet Dishes

Douce ame

Take gode Cowe mylke and do it in a pot. take parsel. sawge. ysope. saueray and ooþer gode herbes. hewe hem and do hem in the mylke and seeþ hem. take capouns half yrosted and smyte hem on pecys and do þerto pynes and hony clarified. salt it and colour it with safroun an serue it forth.

Sweet dish (my translation)

Take good cow's milk and put it in a pot. Take parsley, sage, hyssop, savory and other good herbs. Chop them and put them in milk and simmer them. Take half-roasted capons and chop them into pieces and thereto pine nuts and clarified honey. Salt it and colour it with saffron and serve it forth.[72]

Moroccan mint tea

Put a scant 1 Tbsp of long-leaved green Chinese tea in a teapot. Cover with boiling water, stir, and discard water immediately. Then fill the teapot with fresh mint leaves, or ⅔ cup loose, dried mint leaves, and fill the teapot with boiling water. Add 8 sugar lumps and 1½ tsp of orange-flower water. Let this infuse for 3 or 4 minutes, stir well, and serve in thick glasses.[73]

Doughnuts were very popular it seems in sixteenth-century Transylvania if the Prince of Transylvania's court cookbook, *The Science of Cooking*, is anything to go by. This volume of recipes contains at least ten variations of these delightful dough balls, which would actually have looked a lot more like very solid choux buns. The numerous variations published in this manuscript often come with instructions for replicating a previous method and simply adding an alternative filling; then when you find the original method, you realize you then need to go to another recipe to establish the technique and so on. To make matters easier, I have taken the basic doughnut recipe, combined it with the 'doughnut baking pan' instructions and then woven in the directions to make the sage doughnuts accordingly. As the translation was ever so slightly confusing, here is my modified final recipe for Transylvanian sage doughnuts from the Prince of Transylvania's master chef:

Transylvanian sage doughnuts

Whip some eggs in cold milk; if you want to make enough for one table, twenty eggs will be enough, add lots of flour. Add salt and saffron. Wash and chop some fresh sage and add it to the dough. You need a fairly dense dough. Find a baking pan (made of iron or wood and soaked in butter), put a little butter into it, then pour the batter into the pan and bake it. Once baked, put it on a clean table, slice the crust. Slice the dough into cubes, but not all of it. Find a big enough pan. Have enough dough, for this doughnut will become

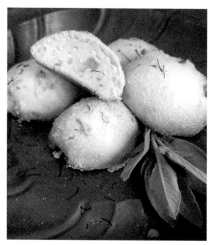

Transylvanian sage doughnuts. (*Emma Kay*)

big. Don't boil the butter, just melt it; have lots of butter, for doughnuts require this. While cooking, put some butter onto it with your spoon. Once the dough is starting to become bigger, put it on the fire again, put butter on it, and wait for it to cook, but keep putting butter onto it. Keep adding butter and rotating. Serve hot and cover in sugar.[74]

My modernized version (makes 20):
50g butter and extra to baste
Caster sugar to dust
220g strong white flour (or enough until a stiff mixture forms)
2 eggs lightly beaten.
150ml milk
1 tsp salt
A pinch of saffron
3 small washed and chopped sage leaves

1. Preheat oven to 220°C/ 200°C fan/gas mark 7.
2. Heat the butter and milk in a saucepan until the butter has melted.
3. Remove from the heat and quickly add the flour, salt, saffron and chopped sage leaves.
4. Beat thoroughly until it comes together. Leave to cool.
5. Beat in the eggs or mix in a food processor, a little at a time. You are looking to achieve a dense cake mixture consistency, that will stand when dropped into balls.
6. Grease a baking tray with butter and blob dessertspoonfuls of the mixture onto the tray. Cook on the middle shelf for between 10–15 minutes, until slightly browned and firm when tapped on the underside.
7. Remove from the oven and baste with melted butter and sugar while still hot.
8. Cool on a wire rack. These little balls could be served with syrup or other sweet sauces of your choice.

Many Islamic sweet dishes contain mint, as with the recipe below for mint syrup, which was taken for medicinal purposes:

Syrup of mint

Take mint and basil, citron and cloves, a handful of each, and cook all this in water [and] cover until its substance comes out, and add the clear part of it to a *ratl* [about 1 pound] of sugar. Then add an *ûqiya* [about 38g] of flower of cloves, and cook all this until a syrup is made. Its benefits: it frees bodies that suffer from phlegm, and cuts phlegmatic urine, fortifies the liver and the stomach, and cheers it a great deal; in this it is admirable.[75]

Marjoram with sugar was once regarded as a useful combination to fight head colds, stomach issues, liver disorders and even heart disease; marjoram conserve was favoured throughout the eighteenth and nineteenth centuries. Here is John Nott's recipe of 1723:

Conserve of marjoram

Take the tops and tenderest part of sweet marjoram, bruise it well in a wooden mortar or bowl; take double the weight of fine sugar, boil it with marjoram-water till it is as thick as syrup, then put in your beaten marjoram.[76]

Biscuits and Confection

Medicines throughout history have been blended into more palatable forms to make confection, including chocolates, comfits, lozenges and 'drops' – anything to sweeten, flavour and make a remedy more appealing to general consumers. We can all relate to Mary Poppins's chant 'A spoonful of sugar helps the medicine go down.'

In fact, the word 'confection' itself originally meant mixing something together, from the Latin *conficere*. As herbs were medicinal, they played a significant role in early pharmaceutical confection and other sweetmeats, 'cakes' and biscuits.

Syrups were another way of preserving both the taste and goodness of fruits, flowers and herbs, which were then used to accompany desserts or as generic sweeteners. Today we seem enamoured with syrups far less than we were in the past, remaining faithful to key favourites like golden syrup, maple syrup and chocolate syrup, none of which have a particularly strong British heritage. William Jarrin's, *The Italian Confectioner* of the early 1800s, lists some fifteen different syrups, several of which were herbal.

The jujube is a type of red Chinese date which was once highly favoured in Spain, Italy and France. Often made into a sort of gum pastille, the word jujube eventually became a generic term for all jelly-like pastilles made using a mix of natural gum Arabic, sugar and flavourings, popular right up to today.

The following is a Victorian recipe for Spanish liquorice jujubes:

1 lb gum Arabic
14 oz of sugar
2 oz Spanish liquorice dissolved in hot water and afterwards strained clean

First prepare the gum and boil it with the sugar as directed in the preceding article (soak the gum in 1 pint of tepid water. Place the soaked, strained gum into a sugar boiler with the sugar, boil and reduce it). When reduced by boiling to the small pearl degree, incorporate the prepared Spanish liquorice with it, remove the scum from the surface and finish the jujubes in the manner indicated above. Cast the jujubes in starch powder [corn starch] and lay in a box.[77]

Caraway comfit

According to John Gerard, 'The seeds [of carraway], confected or made with sugar into comfits, are very good for the stomache, they help digestion, provoke urine, asswage and dissolve all windiness.'[78] Comfits represent one of the oldest and simplest forms of confectionery using sugar. A series of Victorian comfit recipes can be found in J. M. Sanderson's *The Complete Cook*, including the basic carraway variety which initially achieved popularity during the sixteenth century.

Common carraways

Sift the seeds and warm them in a pan. Have some gum Arabic dissolved, throw in a ladleful, and rub them well about the pan with the hand until dry, dusting them with flour. Give them three of four coatings in this manner, and then a charge of sugar, until they are about one half the required size. Dry them for a day, give then two or three coatings of gum and flour, finish them by giving three or four charges of sugar, and dry them. These are made about the size of Bath caraways [probably a

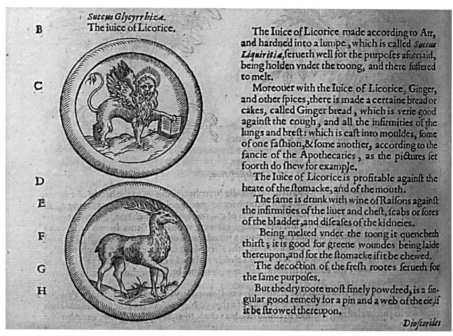

Succus Glycyrrhizæ.
The iuice of Licorice.

The Iuice of Licorice made according to Art, and hardned into a lumpe, which is called *Succus Liquiritia*, serueth well for the purposes aforesaid, being holden vnder the toong, and there suffered to melt.

Moreouer with the Iuice of Licorice, Ginger, and other spices, there is made a certaine bread or cakes, called Ginger bread, which is verie good against the cough, and all the infirmities of the lungs and brest: which is cast into mouldes, some of one fashion,&some another, according to the fancie of the Apothecaries, as the pictures set foorth do shew for example.

The Iuice of Licorice is profitable against the heate of the stomacke, and of the mouth.

The same is drunk with wine of Raisons against the infirmities of the liuer and chest, scabs or sores of the bladder, and diseases of the kidneies.

Being melted vnder the toong it quencheth thirst; it is good for greene woundes being laide thereupon, and for the stomacke if it be chewed.

The decoction of the fresh rootes serueth for the same purposes.

But the dry roote most finely powdred, is a singular good remedy for a pin and a web of the eie, if it be strowed thereupon.

Dioscorides

Liquorice added to gingerbread as noted by Gerard in *The Herball* or *Generall Historie of Plantes*.

couple of centimetres]. Colour parts of them different colours, leaving the greatest portion white.[79]

Gerard also conveyed the medicinal benefits of adding liquorice to gingerbread to aid a variety of respiratory conditions. Gingerbread moulds

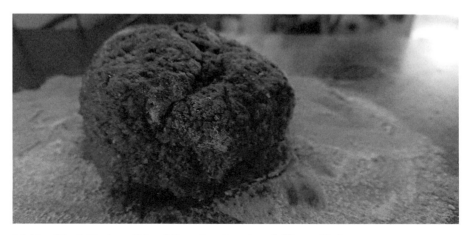

Making Hugh Plat's traditional liquorice gingerbread. (*Emma Kay*)

were crafted by apothecaries who sold this type of liquorice gingerbread in pretty shapes.[80]

The recipe I have included here is from the early 1600s and I have modified it as a slightly more modern interpretation.

Hugh Plat's gingerbread or drie leach

Take three stale manchets and grate them, drie them, and sift them through a fine sieve, then adde unto them one ounce of ginger being beaten and as much cinnamon, one ounce of liquorice and aniseeds being beaten together and searced, halfe a pound of sugar, then boile all these together in a posnet with a quart of claret wine till they come to a stiffe paste with often stirring of it; and when it is stiffe, mold it on a table and so drive it thin, and print it in your moldes, dust your moldes with cinnamon, ginger and liquorice, being mixed together in fine powder. This is your gingerbread served at the court, and in all gentlemens houses at festival times. It is otherwise called drie Leach.[81]

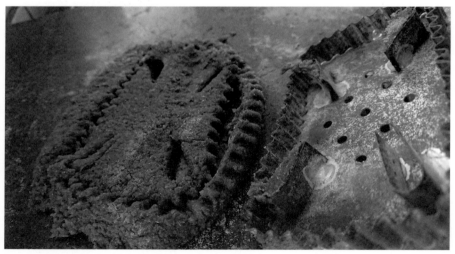

Hugh Plat's traditional liquorice gingerbread. (*Emma Kay*)

Plat's is a no-bake gingerbread recipe, but you could bake it to make it slightly more appetizing. Note that the 'Leach' was a type of medieval sweetmeat, shaped and moulded into decorative treats or sliced into strips. So drie Leach, was simply dried sweetmeats.

My version
100g breadcrumbs
2 tsp ginger
1 tsp cinnamon
1 tsp liquorice root powder (you can purchase this from health food shops, specialist food shops or easily online)
½ tsp aniseed
50g caster sugar
100ml red wine

1. Put the breadcrumbs into a small non-stick saucepan. Add the ginger, cinnamon, liquorice, aniseed, and sugar. Stir well. Pour in the red wine.
2. Heat the mixture on a mid to low setting and it will gradually form a stiff dough. The longer it cooks the stiffer the dough. When it comes together in a firm ball remove from the pan and set aside.
3. Dust a clean board with some cinnamon, ginger and liquorice powder.
4. The dough will be quite sticky, but I found it malleable enough to roll. It helps to dust the rolling pin the same way as the board.
5. You can roll the dough into whatever thickness you like, before casting it into patterned moulds if you have them, or cutting shapes from it with a biscuit cutter. Leave to dry naturally or bake at 180°C for 10–20 minutes depending on the thickness of your dough.

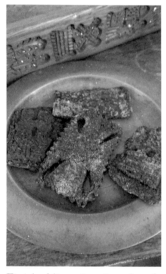

Finished liquorice gingerbread. (*Emma Kay*)

Suckets were typically sweetmeats made using the rind or whole of the fruit, preserved in sugar. During the latter part of the 1500s the word also included other candied foods, from vegetables to nuts. The recipe below is for dried suckets. Wet suckets were cooked in sugar and then preserved in jars, along with their syrup.

Candy suckets of oranges, lemons, citrons and angelica
Take, and boil them in fair water tender, and shift them in three boilings, six or seven times, to take away their bitterness, then put them into as much Sugar as will cover them, and so let them boil a walm or two, then take them out, and dry them in a warm Oven as hot as Manchet, and being dry boil the Sugar to a Candy height, and so cast your Oranges into the hot Sugar, and take them out again suddenly, and then lay them upon a lattice of Wyer or the bottom of a Sieve in a warm Oven after the bread is drawn, still warming the Oven till it be dry, and they will be well candied.[82]

Peppermint drops
Squeeze three or four lemons into a bason, and mix some powdered sugar with the juice, the sugar must be sifted through a lawn sieve; make it of a proper thickness, and put some oil of peppermint in with it, as much as you think proper to your palate; make it of a proper thickness with sugar, put it in a saucepan and dry it over the fire, stirring it with a wooden spoon for five minutes, then drop them off a knife on your writing paper, the same size as the last receipt mentions, and let them stand till they are cold, and they will come off easily, then put them in your papered box.[83]

Wormwood syrup

> 1 oz wormwood
> 1 lb sugar
> Make nearly a pint of the infusion of wormwood; add to it a pound of loaf-sugar; clarify it, and boil it to a pearl; when cold bottle it.

Jarrin's notes for clarifying and making a pearl
To Clarify loaf-sugar – Break the sugar you want into a copper pan, which will hold a third more than the required quantity; put about half a pint of water to every pound of sugar, and beat up some whites of eggs with it: one is sufficient for six pounds of sugar. Put it on the fire, and when it rises in boiling, throw in a little cold water … Let it rise three times without skimming it; the fourth time skim it well, throwing in a little cold water each time, till the white scum ceases to rise; then strain it through a sieve, cloth-strainer, or a flannel bag.

A pearl – When you separate your thumb and finger, and the thread (of sugar) reaches without breaking, from one to the other, it is the small pearl; if the finger and thumb be stretched to their utmost extent, and the thread remain unbroken, it is the large pearl.[84]

Liquorice paste

Scrape and bruise a quarter of a pound of liquorice-root, and boil it in a little water till it is much reduced; let it stand to settle, and pour it clear off, and dissolve it in half an ounce of gum-dragon: when thoroughly dissolved, sift it in a linen bag, and mix sugar with it till it is brought to the consistence of paste; then cut it into what flowers of designs you think proper.[85]

Drinks

Just as sweetened confection puts a positive spin on prescribed remedies, tonics, tinctures, 'waters', wines and all manner of other drinks helped achieve a similar goal. During the nineteenth century herb teas were frequently taken for all manner of complaints from tiredness to colds. Mugwort was used to flavour drinks as far back as the early Iron Age. At one stage in the 1800s the wide use of chicory as a coffee substitute led to all foreign imports being suspended. People just started growing it in England instead.

The *Florentine Codex* of 1552 recommends an Aztec concoction of the skinned, ground and boiled root of tlacoxiloxochitl, which is a species of vanilla, mixed with honey for a bad cough. This is one mixture that I wouldn't actually flinch at trying. The same drink is recommended daily before meals, for anyone who spits blood.[86]

Purl

Purl is basically ale infused with wormwood and other herbs. It seems to have first made an appearance around the beginning of the 1700s, but there were plenty of drinks being made with wormwood long before, as it was a herb regularly used to soothe the stomach, providing remedies aplenty for the ancient Egyptians and Greeks.

In Britain wormwood became a popular way to spice up mead, something we inherited from the Romans, but in early medieval times it was also believed the herb could protect individuals from witchcraft and necromancy. Excessive amounts of wormwood can be toxic – but you would need to consume an awful lot of it! Its flavour is very bitter and as such it appears as a metaphor in numerous historic texts from Shakespeare to Roald Dahl. Today wormwood is still used in the production of the potent Swiss/French alcoholic drink, absinthe; the word is derived from both the Latin and Greek words for wormwood.

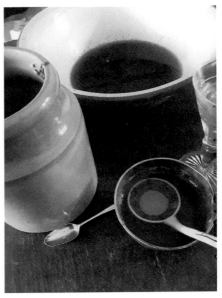

Making traditional purl. (*Emma Kay*)

The following is my recreated amalgamation of two different recipes taken from S. Moor's 1812 edition of *The Publican's Friend, and Sure Guide to Do Well* and *Mackenzie's Five Thousand Receipts in All the Useful and Domestic Arts* of 1851:

57g of gentian root cut into small pieces
28g of wormwood
28g of horseradish
28g of orange peel rinds
28g of lemon peel rinds

Put the gentian root into a cask. Or in this case a stone jar. Bruise all the other ingredients in a mortar, then add them to the gentian root. Add 2¼ litres of mild beer. Stir. (One recipe stipulates repeating the process all over again over ten days, while the other suggests just leaving it all to infuse for several months before straining.)

According to the late Scottish folklorist, political activist and author Florence Marian McNeill, this recipe for Highland bitters was 'very old' when noting it down in the 1920s.

Highland bitters, from the Scots kitchen
Gentian root, coriander seed, quarter of an ounce of chamomile flower, quarter of an ounce of cinnamon stick, and half an ounce of cloves. Bruise all together. Put in an earthenware jar, empty two bottles of whisky over it, cover so that the jar is airtight, and let it stand for about ten days. Strain and bottle. More whisky may be added to the flavouring materials, which remain good for a long time.[87]

Tredure was a type of caudle, which the next recipe actually refers to in the method. A caudle (from the Latin *caldus*, for warm) was a hot thick and sweet drink often prepared with ale or wine. It was almost certainly served as a strengthening drink, one often given to the sick and infirm.

Tredure
Take Brede and grate it. make a lyre of rawe ayrenn and do þerto Safroun and powdour douce. and lye it up with gode broth. and make it as a Cawdel. and do þerto a lytel verious.[88]

Tredure (my translation)
Take bread and grate it, make a lyre (thickener) of raw eggs, and add to it saffron and sweet spices and mix it up with good broth and make it as a caudle. Add a little verjuice (see recipe earlier in this chapter).

Metheglin is an ancient, flavoured mead, mead being one of the earliest of all alcoholic beverages in Britain, brewed by Celtic Druids. Metheglin, which actually means medicine, from the Welsh word *meddyglyn*, as this type of mead largely contained herbs, leaves or/and flowers, has never found fashion in contemporary society. Sir Kenelme Digbie wrote a whole section on metheglin in his 1669 book, *The Closet of the Eminently Learned Sir Kenelme Digbie Knight, Opened*, which included the following recipe:

A receipt to make a tun of metheglin
Take two handfuls of Dock [*alias* wild carrot] a reasonable burthen of Saxifrage, Wild-sage, Blew-button, Scabious, Bettony, Agrimony, Wild-marjoram, of each a reasonable burthen; Wild-thyme a Peck, Roots, and all. All these are to be gathered in the fields, between the two Lady days in Harvest. The Garden-herbs are these; Bay-leaves, and Rosemary, of each two handfuls; a Sieveful of Avens, and as much Violet-leaves:

A handful of Sage; three handfuls of Sweet-Marjoram, Three Roots of young Borrage, leaves and all, that hath not born seed; Two handfuls of Parsley-roots, and all that hath not born Seed. Two Roots of Elecampane that have not seeded: Two handfuls of Fennel that hath not seeded: A peck of Thyme; wash and pick all your herbs from filth and grass: Then put your field herbs first into the bottom of a clean Furnace, and lay all your Garden-herbs thereon; then fill your Furnace with clean water, letting your herbs seeth, till they be so tender, that you may easily slip off the skin of your Field-herbs, and that you may break the roots of your Garden-herbs between your Fingers. Then lade forth your Liquor, and set it a cooling. Then fill your Furnace again with clear water to these Herbs, and let them boil a quarter of an hour. Then put it to your first Liquor, filling the Furnace, until you have sufficient to fill your Tun. Then as your Liquor begins to cool, and is almost cold, set your servants to temper Honey and wax in it, Combs, and all, and let them temper it well together, breaking the Combes very small; let their hands and nails be very clean; and when you have tempered it very well together, cleanse it through a cleansing sieve into another clean vessel; The more Honey you have in your Liquor, the stronger it will be. Therefore to know, when it is strong enough, take two New-laid eggs, when you begin to cleanse, and put them in whole into the bottome of your cleansed Liquor; And if it be strong enough, it will cause the Egge to ascend upward, and to be on the top as broad as sixpence; if they do not swim on the top; put more.[89]

The aromatic Southern European herb balm, or as we know it better now as lemon balm, was extremely popular in the nineteenth century. Its fragrant lemon flavour made it a popular choice for teas and wine, to relieve fevers and diseases of the lungs. It was even used to coax bees into their hives. The subsequent recipe for balm wine was published in the 1849 edition of *The British Wine-maker and Domestic Brewer*:

Balm wine
This is made by pouring boiling water on the leaves of balm, after they have been separated from their stalks. One bushel of leaves to eight gallons of water is employed. When the water has been poured on them, they are well mixed up and allowed to remain for twenty-four hours. They are then strained and the liquor measured and weighed by the saccharometer. The gravity of this wine need not exceed 110, which is to be made up

with loaf sugar. If it is properly made, it is a remarkably soft, pleasant wine, and improves greatly by keeping. I have drunk some of this wine many years old, and I really was at a loss to give it a name.[90]

There are over sixty varieties of sage, but only a couple of these are native to England.

To make sage wine

Boil twenty-six quarts [1 quart is c. 1 litre, so this would be 26 litres] of spring water a quarter of an hour and when it is blood-warm, put into it twenty-five pounds (14 pounds in a stone – so this would be around 2 stone or 12 kilograms (as there are 6 kilograms in 1 stone) of malaga raisins, picked, rubbed and shred, with near half a bushel [4 gallons – about 16 kilograms] of red sage shred, and a porringer of ale yeast; stir all well together, and let it stand in a tub, covered warm, six or seven days, stirring it once a day; then strain it off, and put it in a runlet [cask]; let it work three or four days, and then stop it up; when it has stood six or seven days, put in a quart or two of malaga sack; when it is fine, bottle it. [91]

Following is an adapted version of the recipe above. If you want to make less, simply reduce the quantities of all the ingredients accordingly.

Heat 26 litres of water until tepid. Add 12 kilograms of raisins, 16 kilograms of red sage, 6 grams of Saccharomyces cerevisiae yeast (the best for winemaking). Stir well, cover for about a week in a covered tub, stirring every day. Transfer to a wooden casket, or stone jar. Leave for three days, seal it and leave for a further six or seven days. Add 1–2 litres of sweet, Spanish wine, strain and bottle.

This recipe below using hyssop was said to make a good wine that was useful for griping, chills or fevers, as well as with helping to induce a woman's monthly menstrual cycle.

Hyssop wine

'The best hyssop wine is that which is made from Cilician hyssop … Put one pound of bruised hyssop leaves (wrapped in a thin linen cloth) into nine gallons of must (a freshly crushed fruit juice – usually grape) and also put in small stones so that the bundle subsides to the bottom. After forty days strain it and put it in another jar. It is good for disorders in the chest, side, and lungs and for old coughs and asthma. It is diuretic, good for griping and the periodical chills of fevers, and it induces the menstrual flow'.[92]

Benedictine liqueur is one of the oldest commercial liqueurs predominantly made with herbs. It was first produced during the Renaissance in Normandy, incorporating cognac with a variety of nearly thirty different herbs and spices, including thyme, coriander, hyssop and angelica. Macerated and distilled over many years in separate batches, before being aged in oak casks, the various herbs and spices were then brought together as one blend. The original recipe, or as it was once known, the elixir of life, is said to have been forged by Dom Bernardo Vincelli from the Benedictine Abbey in Fécamp and disappeared when the abbey closed during the French Revolution, before being rediscovered and trademarked in the nineteenth century.[93]

Of course, this is the story of wine merchant Alexandre le Grand, who rediscovered Benedictine, but may well have simply made up any old concoction to sell. Whatever the real narrative of the recipe is, the process of making Benedictine liqueur remains a closely guarded secret.

Here is a cocktail from the 1870s called the Moselle Cup (a wine produced along the Moselle River), which contains a shot of the old elixir itself.

Moselle Cup

To 1 bottle of Moselle, still or sparkling, add 1 bottle of Vichy, seltzer or soda water, 3 tangerine oranges cut in slices, some sprigs of borage or Woodroffe, 1 glass of Benedictine liqueur, powdered sugar candy to taste, some pieces of pure block ice. Should the bouquet of the wine be flat, a few bruised Muscatel grapes may be added.[94]

Saloop

I am aware that orchids are not herbs, but I have included other flowers of note in this book, under this generic title. Some flowers have traditionally been used in herbal medicines and as culinary additions in salads and as garnishes for hundreds of years. As such, I felt I had to include saloop here.

The subsequent method of preparation for the saloop powder was outlined by a Mr Moult in the Philosophical Transactions of the Royal Society in the 1880s, before being published in *Cassell's Dictionary* and includes detailed instructions, using English, opposed to traditional Turkish orchid bulbs:

The best time to gather the roots is when the seed is forming and the stalk [is] going to fall; for then the new bulb, of which the salep is made, is arrived to its full size, and may be known from the old one, whose strength is then spent by the preceding germination, by a white bud rising from the top of it, which is the germ of the plant of the succeeding ear. This new root, being separated from the stalk, is to be washed in water, and a fine thin skin that covers it to be taken off with a small brush; or, by dipping in hot water, it will come off with a coarse linen cloth. When a sufficient quantity of the roots is thus cleaned, they are to be spread on a tin plate, and set into an oven heated to the degree of a bred oven, where they are to remain six, eight or ten minutes, in which time they will have lost their milky whiteness, and have acquired a transparency like that of a horn, but without being diminished in size. When they are arrived at this state, they may be removed to another room to dry and harden, which will be done in a few days; or they must be finished in a very slow heat in a few hours.

Cassell's published a recipe alongside this:

Take a dessertspoonful of the powder of saloop, and add it to a pint of boiling water. Keep stirring till the preparation becomes of the consistence of jelly, then add white wine and sugar to taste.[95]

Notes

Introduction
1. *September*, Helen Hunt Jackson (1892).
2. Northcote, R., *The Book of Herbs* (John Lane, London & New York, 1903).
3. World Health Organization, *Legal Status of Traditional Medicine and Complementary/Alternative Medicine: Worldwide Review*. (WHO, Geneva, 2001).
4. Harvey, J. H., *Garden Plants of around 1525: The Fromond List*, Garden History, Vol. 17, No. 2 (1989).
5. Landsberg, S, *The Medieval Garden* (University of Toronto Press, 2003) 79–81.
6. Gerard, J., *The Herball or Generall Historie of Plantes* (John Norton, London, 1597).
7. Murrey, T. J., *Salads and Sauces*, (Frederick A. Stokes, New York, 1884) 204.
8. Rhode, E., *The Old English Herbals* (Minerva Press, London, 1974).
9. Boswell, J., (ed.), *English Botany, or Coloured Figures of British Plants* (George Bell & Sons, London, 1878).
10. Da Silva, Z., *The Herb in History, Mysteries and Crafts* (Cambridge Scholars Publishing, Newcastle upon Tyne, 2017) 10.
11. Shou-zhong, Y., *A Translation of the Shen Nong Ben Cao Jing* (Blue Poppy Press, USA, 1998).
12. Da Silva, Z., *The Herb in History, Mysteries and Crafts* (Cambridge Scholars Publishing, Newcastle upon Tyne, 2017) 11.
13. Bottéro, J., 'The Culinary Tablets at Yale', *Journal of the American Oriental Society*, Vol. 107, No. 1 (1987).
14. Veenker, R. A., *The Biblical Archaeologist*, Vol. 44, No .4 (1981).
15. Walcott Emmart, E., *Concerning the Badianus Manuscript, an Aztec Herbal, 'Codex Barberini, Latin 241'* (The Smithsonian Institute, Washington, 1935).
16. *The Japanese Pharmacopoeia*, 17th edition (2016), www.mhlw.go.jp/file/06-Seisakujouhou-11120000-Iyakushokuhinkyoku/JP17_REV_1.pdf (accessed 3 June 2021).
17. Mahomoodally, M., *Traditional Medicines in Africa: An Appraisal of Ten Potent African Medicinal Plants* (Hindawi, 2013), www.who.int/mediacentre/news/releases/release38/en/ (accessed 30 May 2021).
18. Britten, W., *Art Magic, or Mundane, Sub-mundane and Super-mundane Spiritism* (New York, 1876).
19. Da Silva, Z., *The Herb in History, Mysteries and Crafts* (Cambridge Scholars Publishing, Newcastle Upon Tyne, 2017) 18–20.
20. *A History of Magic and Experimental Science* Vol. 1 (Columbia University Press, New York & London, 1923) 74.
21. *A History of Magic and Experimental Science* Vol. 1 (Columbia University Press, New York & London, 1923) 19.
22. *The Philosophy of Natural Magic* (Jazzybee Verlag Jurgen Beck, 2014).

23. Thomas, K., *Religion, and the Decline of Magic* (Penguin, London, 2003) 648.
24. Cockayne, T. O., *Leechdoms, Wortcunning and Starcraft,* Vol. 1 (Cambridge University Press, 1864).
25. Thomas, K., *Religion, and the Decline of Magic* (Penguin, London, 2003).
26. Britten, W., *Art Magic, or Mundane, Sub-mundane and Super-mundane Spiritism* (New York, 1876) 407.
27. Green, M., *The Trotula, An English Translation of the Medieval compendium of Women's Medicine* (University of Pennsylvania Press, 2002) 39.
28. Rowland B, *Medieval Guide to Women's Health* (Kent University Press, Kent, Ohio, 1981) 11
29. Forbes, T. R, *The Midwife, and the Witch* (AMS Press, 1982) 117.
30. Summers, Montague (trans), *The Malleus Maleficarum* (1928) www.sacred-texts. com/pag/mm/index.htm (accessed 22 March 2021).
31. WHO, *Global Report on Traditional and Complementary Medicine* (WHO, Luxembourg, 2019).
32. *Herbal medicine market size and forecast, by product (tablets & capsules, powders, extracts), by indication (digestive disorders, respiratory disorders, blood disorders), and trend analysis, 2014–2024* (Market Research Report, Hexa Research2017) www. hexaresearch.com/research-report/global-herbal-medicine-market (accessed 2 March 2021).

Chapter 1

1. Shakespeare, W., *Romeo and Juliet, Act V, Scene 1* (Stanley Thornes, 2014).
2. BBC News, 30 March 2015, *1,000-year-old onion and garlic eye remedy kills MRSA* www.bbc.co.uk/news/uk-england-nottinghamshire-32117815 (accessed 10 June 2021).
3. Rawcliffe, C., *Delectable Sightes and Fragrant Smelles: Gardens and Health in Late Medieval and Early Modern England.* Garden History, Vol. 36, No. 1 (2008).
4. Delany, P., *Constantinus Africanus' 'De Coitu'* A Translation, The Chaucer Review, Vol. 4, No. 1 (Penn State University Press).
5. Thompson, C. J., *The Apothecary in England from the Thirteenth to the Close of the Sixteenth Century* (Proceedings of the Royal Society of Medicine, London, 1915).
6. British Newspaper Archive *Bradford Observer* (25 February, 1943).
7. Curran, R., *A Bewitched Land. Ireland's Witches* (The O'Brien Press, Ireland, 2012).
8. *Halsbury's Statutes of England* Vol. 21 (Butterworths, London,1970).
9. Chaucer, G., *The Canterbury Tales*, (Oxford University Press, Oxford &New York, 2011).
10. Harvey, J., Daniel, Henry, *A Scientific Gardener of the Fourteenth Century*, Garden History, Vol. 15, No. 2 (1987).
11. Ibid.
12. Turner, W., *The First and Seconde Partes of the Herbal of William Turner* (Arnold Birckman, 1568)
13. Smith, M., *William Turner (C. 1508–1568): Physician, Botanist and Theologian* (Journal of Medical Biology, 1999).
14. *Speeches Delivered to Queen Elizabeth, on Her Visit to Giles Brudges, Lord Chandos , at Sudeley Castle , in Gloucestershire.* (Johnson & Warwick, London, 1815).
15. Pett, D. E., *The Cornwall Gardens Guide* (Alison Hodge, 2006) 246.

16. Isely, D., *One Hundred and One Botanists* (Purdue University Press, 2002) 47.

17. Williamson, G. C., *Lady Anne Clifford, Countess of Dorset, Pembroke & Montgomery, 1590-1676. Her life, letters, and work, extracted from all the original documents available, many of which are here printed for the first time* (Kendal Titus Wilson & Son, 1922) 38.

18. Leong, E., *Herbals She Peruseth': Reading Medicine in Early Modern England*, Renaissance Studies, Vol. 28, No. 4 (2014).

19. Woolf, J., *Women's Business: 17th Century Female Pharmacists* (Science History Institute, 2009).

20. Baynes, R. H., (ed.), *The Churchman's Shilling Magazine and Family Treasury*, Vol. 16, (Houlston & Sons, London, 1874) 141–4.

21. Parkinson, A., *Nature's Alchemist* (Francis Lincoln Ltd, London, 2007).

22. Parkinson, J., *Paradisi in sole paradisus terrestris* (Methuen & Co, 1904) 477.

23. Parkinson, A., *Nature's Alchemist*, (Francis Lincoln Ltd, London, 2007).

24. Ibid., 8.

25. Woolley, B., *The Herbalist. Nicholas Culpeper and the Fight for Medical Freedom* (Harper Collins, London, 2012).

26. Olav, T., *Nicholas Culpeper: English Physician and Astrologer* (Palgrave Macmillan, London, 1992).

27. Sellar, A. M., *Bede's Ecclesiastical History of England, A Revised Translation* (George Bell & Sons, London, 1907) 190.

28. Brooke, E., *Women Healers Through History*, (Aeon Books, 2020) 35.

29. Whaley, L., *Women, and the Practice of Medical care in Early Modern Europe, 1400–1800* (Palgrave Macmillan, London, 2011) 102.

30. Pelling, M., White, F., in *Physicians and Irregular Medical Practitioners in London 1550–1640 Database* (London, 2004), *British History Online*, www.british-history.ac.uk/no-series/london-physicians/1550-1640/ (accessed 26 March 2021).

31. Levack, B. P., *Witchcraft in Scotland* (Garland Publishing Inc., New York & London, 1992) 18.

32. Pelling, M & White, F., 'JACKSON, Elizabeth', in *Physicians and Irregular Medical Practitioners in London 1550-1640 Database* (London, 2004), *British History Online*, www.british-history.ac.uk/no-series/london-physicians/1550-1640/jackson-elizabeth (accessed 26 March 2021).

33. Leong, E., *Making Medicines in the Early Modern Household*, Bulletin of the History of Medicine, Vol. 82, No. 1 (2008), www.jstor.org/stable/44448509?readnow=1&refreqid=excelsior%3Afb4a0bd167d8336ff464b10fe1473f04&seq=19#page_scan_tab_contents (accessed 14 April, 2021).

34. Raven, C. E., *John Ray Naturalist: His Life and Works* (Cambridge University Press, Cambridge, London, New York, Melbourne, New Rochelle, Sydney, 1950) 67.

35. Isely, D., *One Hundred and One Botanists* (Purdue University Press, 2002) 68.

36. Rousseau, G, *The Notorious Sir John Hill* (Lehigh University Press, 2012).

37. Brown, P. C., *Essex Witches* (The History Press, 2014)

38. Monod, P. K., *Solomon's Secret Arts.* (Yale University Press, New Haven & London, 2013) 196.

39. Davies, O., *Witchcraft, Magic, and Culture, 1736–1951* (Manchester University Press, 1999) 220.

40. British Newspaper Archive *Lancashire Evening Post* (15 August, 1933).

41. British Newspaper Archive *Lancashire Evening Post* (25 July, 1957).

42. Madge, B, *Elizabeth Blackwell: The Forgotten Herbalist?* (Wiley Online Library, 2003).

43. Ibid.

44. Ibid.

45. *Notes and Queries* Vol. 5, January–June (John Francis, London, 1876).

46. Sloane, H., *An Account of a Most Efficacious Medicine for Soreness, Weakness, and Several Other Distempers of the Eyes* (London, 1745).

47. Ibid., 5.

48. Denham, Alison M., *Herbal Medicine in Nineteenth Century England: The Career of John Skelton* (University of York, 2013).

49. Atkinson, T, *Napier's History of Herbal Healing* (Creative Print&Design, Wales, 2003) 50–1.

50. Minter, Sue, *The Well-Connected Gardener* (Book Guild Publishing, 2010).

51. Amherst, A., *A History of Gardening in England* (Bernard Quaritch, Lonon, 1895) 103–4.

52. *Duncan Napier's Diary Records*, https://amp.ww.en.freejournal.org/13497030/1/duncan-napier.html (accessed 20 April, 2021).

53. Vickery, R., *Vickery's Folk Flora* (Weidenfeld & Nicolson, 2019).

54. Griggs, B., *Helpful Herbs for Health and Beauty* (2008) 36.

55. *Duncan Napier's Diary Records* https://amp.ww.en.freejournal.org/13497030/1/duncan-napier.html (accessed 20 April, 2021).

56. Stobart, A., *Household Medicine in Seventeenth-Century England* (Bloomsbury Academic, London, 2016) 75.

57. The Old Bailey, Ref: t18261026-215.

58. British Newspaper Archive *Sheffield Daily Telegraph* (29 November, 1855).

59. British Newspaper Archive *Edinburgh Evening News* (7 January, 1884).

60. The Old Bailey, Ref: t18481023-2442.

61. Marland, H., *Medicine and Society in Wakefield and Huddersfield 1780-1870*, (Cambridge University Press, 1987) 241.

62. Pelling, M., White, F., 'ACTOUR, John', in *Physicians and Irregular Medical Practitioners in London 1550–1640 Database* (London, 2004), *British History Online*, www.british-history.ac.uk/no-series/london-physicians/1550-1640/actour-john (accessed 26 March 2021).

63. Pelling, M., White, F., 'ANTHONY, Francis', in *Physicians and Irregular Medical Practitioners in London 1550–1640 Database* (London, 2004), *British History Online*, www.british-history.ac.uk/no-series/london-physicians/1550-1640/anthony-francis (accessed 26 March 2021) .

64. Pelling, M., White, F., 'AUDLING, Edward', in *Physicians and Irregular Medical Practitioners in London 1550–1640 Database* (London, 2004), *British History Online*, www.british-history.ac.uk/no-series/london-physicians/1550-1640/audling-edward (accessed 26 March 2021).

65. Pelling, M., White, F., 'GLORIANA, Susanna', in *Physicians and Irregular Medical Practitioners in London 1550–1640 Database* (London, 2004), *British History Online*, www.british-history.ac.uk/no-series/london-physicians/1550-1640/gloriana-susanna (accessed 26 March 2021).

66. Pelling, M., White, F., 'DESILAR, Matthew', in *Physicians and Irregular Medical Practitioners in London 1550–1640 Database* (London, 2004), *British History Online*, www.british-history.ac.uk/no-series/london-physicians/1550-1640/desilar-matthew (accessed 26 March 2021).

67. British Newspaper Archive *Bellshill Speaker* (28 December 1901).

68. Sheppard, E., *Memorials of St. James's Palace, Volume 1* (Longmans, Green & Co., London, 1894) 145.

69. Strickland, A., *Lives of the Queens of England* (George Bell & Sons, London, 1884).

70. Furnivall, F. J., *Harrisons Description of England in Shakespeare's Youth* (The New Shakespeare Society, London, 1877) 73.

71. Pegge, S., *Curialia miscellanea* (J. Nichols, Son & Bentley, London, 1818) 44.

72. Plat, Hugh, *The Garden of Eden* (1653).

73. Keene, D. J, Harding, V., 'St. Pancras Soper Lane 145/30', in *Historical Gazetteer of London Before the Great Fire Cheapside; Parishes of All Hallows Honey Lane, St Martin Pomary, St Mary Le Bow, St Mary Colechurch and St Pancras Soper Lane* (London, 1987), *British History Online*, www.british-history.ac.uk/no-series/london-gazetteer-pre-fire/pp766-767 (accessed 13 March 2021).

74. Knight, C., *London* Vols 1–2 (Charles Knight & Co., London, 1841) 135.

75. Ebsworth, J., (ed)., *The Roxburghe Ballards* (Stephen Austin & Sons, Hertford, 1893).

76. Leong, E., *Making Medicines in the Early Modern Household*, Bulletin of the History of Medicine, Vol. 82, No. 1 (2008), www.jstor.org/stable/44448509?readnow=1&refreqid=excelsior%3Afb4a0bd167d8336ff464b10fe1473f04&seq=19#page_scan_tab_contents (accessed 14 April, 2021).

77. Sheppard, F. H., (ed.) 'Covent Garden Market', in *Survey of London: Volume 36, Covent Garden*, (London, 1970), *British History Online* www.british-history.ac.uk/survey-london/vol36/pp129-150 (accessed 17 June 2021).

78. King, S., Timmins, G., *Making Sense of the Industrial Revolution English Economy and Society 1700–1850* (Manchester University Press, 2001).

79. Spackman, W. F., *An Analysis of the Occupations of the People of the United Kingdom of Great Britain* (William Frederick Spackman, London, 1847).

80. Mayhew, H., *London Labour and the London Poor* Vol. 1 (Griffin, Bohn & Company, London, 1861).

81. Ibid.

82. British Newspaper Archive *Nottingham Journal* (23 October, 1913).

83. Jalkson, L., *Ten Centuries of European Progress* (Sampson Low, Marston & Company Ltd., London, 1893) 47.

84. BBC News, Babbs, H., *London's History of Herbal Treatments* (2011), www.bbc.co.uk/news/uk-england-london-13713424 (accessed 20 June 2021); Hunting, P, *The Worshipful Society of Apothecaries of London* (BMJ Publishing Group, London, 2004); Oxford Botanic Garden, www.obga.ox.ac.uk/1648-collection (accessed 05 April, 2021); *The Apothecaries' Garden* (The History Press, 2000); Foust, C., *Rhubarb. The Wonderous Drug* (Princeton University Press, New Jersey, 1992). Parkinson, S., *A Journal of a Voyage to the South Seas, in His Majesty's Ship The Endeavour* (London, 1773); Kelley, T. M., *Clandestine Marriage. Botany and Romantic Culture* (Johns Hopkins University Press, 2012); North, M., Symonds, J., (ed.) *Recollections of a Happy Life, Being the Autobiography of Marianne North* (Macmillan, New York, 1894).

85. Hunting, P., *The Worshipful Society of Apothecaries of London*, (BMJ Publishing Group, London, 2004).

86. Oxford Botanic Garden,www.obga.ox.ac.uk/1648-collection (accessed 5 April, 2021).

87. Minter, S., *The Well-Connected Gardener* (Book Guild Publishing, 2010).

88. Foust, C., *Rhubarb: The Wonderous Drug* (Princeton University Press, New Jersey, 1992) 116.

89. George, A., *A Banksia Album* (National Library of Australia, 2011) 121.

90. Parkinson, S., *A Journal of a Voyage to the South Seas, in His Majesty's Ship The Endeavour* (London, 1773).

91. Kelley, T, M, *Clandestine Marriage. Botany and Romantic Culture* (Johns Hopkins University Press, 2012).

92. North, M., Symonds, J., (ed.) *Recollections of a Happy Life, Being the Autobiography of Marianne North* (Macmillan, New York, 1894).

93. Sibly, E., *A Key to Physic, and the Occult Sciences* (London, 1795).

94. Creese, M. R. C., Creese, T., *Ladies in the Laboratory III* (The Scarecrow Press, Plymouth, 2010) 7.

95. Brown, P., *Botanical Drawing* (Search Press, 2017).

96. Tansley, A. G., 'Arthur Harry Church. 1865–1937', Obituary Notices of Fellows of the Royal Society, Vol. 2, No. 7 (1939).

Chapter 2

1. Wilde, O., Small, I. (ed.), *The Complete Works of Oscar Wilde* (Oxford University Press, Oxford & New York, 2005).

2. Cunningham, S., *Cunningham's Encyclopaedia of Magical Herbs* (2012).

3. Lecouteux, C., *The High Magic of Talismans and Amulets, Tradition and Craft* (Simon & Schuster, 2014).

4. Hajar, R., The Air of History (Part II) Medicine in the Middle Ages, *History of Medicine* Vol. 13, issue 4 (2012) 158–62.

5. British Newspaper Archive *Belfast News-letter* (25 December 1905).

6. Payne, R. (trans), *Hortulus. De Cultura hortulorum* (Hunt Botanical Library, Pittsburgh, 1966).

7. Spitalfields Life, *The Nine Herb Charm*, https://spitalfieldslife.com/2018/05/15/the-nine-herbs-charm/ (accessed 2 February 2021).

8. Gimassi, R., *Old World Witchcraft* (Weiser Books, San Francisco,2011) 120.

9. Von Störck, Anton, *Observations Upon a Treatise on the Virtues of Hemlock* (J. Meres, London, 1761).

10. Curie, P. H., *Domestic Homoeopathy* (Jesper Harding, Philadelphia, 1839).

11. Jonson, B., Gifford, W. (ed.), *The Works of Ben Jonson with a Biographical Memoir* (George Routledge & Sons, London & New York, 1869).

12. Pennick, N., *Operative Witchcraft* (Destiny Books, Rochester, Vermont, 2019).

13. Lees, E., *The Botanical Looker-out Among the Wild Flowers of the Fields, Woods and Mountains of England and Wales* (Adams & Co., Hamilton, 1851).

14. Cunningham, S., *Cunningham's Encyclopaedia of Magical Herbs* (2012).

15. Dioscorides, P., *De Materia Medica* (IBIDIS Press, South Africa, 2000).

16. Gerard, J., *The Herball or Generall Historie of Plantes*, (John Norton, London, 1597) 848.

17. Cunningham, S., *Cunningham's Encyclopaedia of Magical Herbs* (2012).

18. Folkard, R., *Plant Lore, Legends, and Lyrics: Embracing the Myths, Traditions, Superstitions and Folk-lore of the Plant Kingdom* (S. Low, Marston, Searle & Rivington, New York, 1884).

19. Ibid.

20. Fernie, W. T., *Herbal Simples* (John Wright & Co., Bristol, 1897).
21. Shakespeare, W., *The Oxford Shakespeare: Richard II* (Oxford University Press, Oxford, 2011) 201.
22. Woodville, W., *Medical Botany Containing Systematic and General Descriptions with Plates* (James Phillips, London, 1790).
23. Della Porta, G., *Natural Magick* (John Wright, London, 1669).
24. Thorndike, L., *A History of Magic and Experimental Science,* Vol. 1 (Columbia University Press, New York & London, 1923) 86.
25. Culpeper, N., *Culpeper's Complete Herbal* (J. Gleve & Son, Manchester, 1826).
26. Grieve, Maud, Marshall, M., *A Modern Herbal,* Vol. 1 (Dover Publications, 1971).
27. Cockayne, T. O., *Leechdoms, Wortcunning and Starcraft* Vol. 1 (Cambridge University Press, 1864).
28. Von Nettesheim, H. C., *The Philosophy of Natural Magic* (Jazzybee Verlag Jurgen Beck, 2014).
29. Cunningham, S., *Cunningham's Encyclopaedia of Magical Herbs* (2012) 81.
30. Small, E., *North American Cornucopia* (2013).
31. Kieschnick, J., *The Eminent Monk. Buddhist Ideals in Medieval Chinese Hagiography* (Kuroda Institute, Hawaii, 1997) 24.
32. Leyel, C. F., *Cinquefoil* (Health Research Books, 2007).
33. Cockayne, T. O., *Leechdoms, Wortcunning and Starcraft* Vol. 1 (Cambridge University Press, 1864).
34. Friend, H., *Flowers, and Flower Lore* (W. S. Sonnenschein, 1884).
35. Northcote, R., *The Book of Herbs* (John Lane, London & New York, 1903).
36. Schwemer, D., G. van Buylaere, M. Luukko & T. Abusch, *Corpus of Mesopotamian Anti-Witchcraft Rituals* Vol. 3 (Brill, Leiden & Boston, 2020) 8.
37. Cockayne, T. O., *Leechdoms, Wortcunning and Starcraft* Vol. 1 (Cambridge University Press, 1864) 175.
38. Greene, R., *Quip for an Upstart Courtier* (1592).
39. *A History of Magic and Experimental Science* Vol. 1 (Columbia University Press, New York & London, 1923).
40. Sneddon, A., *Witchcraft and Magic in Ireland* (Palgrave Macmillan 2015).
41. Cunningham, S., *Cunningham's Encyclopaedia of Magical Herbs* (2012).
42. Homer, Fagles, R., Know, B. (eds), *The Odyssey* (Penguin Books, London, 2002).
43. Gerard, J., *The Herball or Generall Historie of Plantes* (John Norton, London, 1597) 145.
44. Folkard, R., *Plant Lore, Legends, and Lyrics: Embracing the Myths, Traditions, Superstitions and Folk-lore of the Plant Kingdom* (S. Low, Marston, Searle & Rivington, New York, 1884) 349.
45. British Newspaper Archive *Edinburgh Evening News* (5 May 1939).
46. Cunningham, S., *Cunningham's Encyclopaedia of Magical Herbs* (2012).
47. Northcote, R., *The Book of Herbs* (John Lane, London & New York, 1903).
48. Cox, N. & Dannehl, K., 'Hearing horn – Hellebore', in *Dictionary of Traded Goods and Commodities 1550–1820* (Wolverhampton, 2007), *British History Online*, www.british-history.ac.uk/no-series/traded-goods-dictionary/1550-1820/hearing-horn-hellebore (accessed 21 June 2021)
49. Powell, R., 'The Magical Flower Used in Invisibility Ointments and Flying Powders', *Sydney Morning Herald* (Sydney, 2021).

50. Cox, N. & Dannehl, K., 'Hemp – Herse', in *Dictionary of Traded Goods and Commodities 1550–1820* (Wolverhampton, 2007), *British History Online*, www.british-history.ac.uk/no-series/traded-goods-dictionary/1550-1820/hemp-herse (accessed 28 June 2021).
51. Gamache, H., *The Magic of Herbs* (Health Research, 1972) 48.
52. Dioscorides, P., *De Materia Medica* (IBIDIS Press, South Africa, 2000).
53. Illes, J., *Pure Magic. A Complete Course in Spellcasting* (Weiser Books, San Francisco, 2007) 111.
54. Dyer, T. F., *The Folklore of Plants* (D. Appleton & Co., New York, 1889).
55. Walafrid, S., *On the Cultivation of Gardens. A Ninth Century Gardening Book* (Ithuriel's Spear, San Francisco, 2009).
56. Folkard, R., *Plant Lore, Legends, and Lyrics: Embracing the Myths, Traditions, Superstitions and Folk-lore of the Plant Kingdom* (S. Low, Marston, Searle & Rivington, New York, 1884)
57. Von Bingen, Hildegard & P. Throop (illus), *Hildegard von Bingen's Physica* (Healing Arts Press, Rochester, 1998) 25.
58. Cockayne, T. O., *Leechdoms, Wortcunning and Starcraft* Vol. 1 (Cambridge University Press, 1864)
59. Ibid.
60. Hartland, E. S., *The Legend of Perseus* (D. Nutt, London, 1894) 154.
61. Lee, M. R., *The Solanaceae II: The Mandrake; in League with the Devil* Vol. 36 (J.R. College of Physicians, Edinburgh, 2006,) 278–85, www.rcpe.ac.uk/journal/issue/journal_36_3/W_Lee_2.pdf (accessed 3 May 2021).
62. Parkinson, J., *A Garden of all Sorts of Pleasant Flowers* (Humfrey Lownes & Robert Young, London, 1629).
63. Simoons, F. J., *Plants of Life, Plants of Death* (University of Wisconsin Press, 1998) 119.
64. Folkard, R., *Plant Lore, Legends, and Lyrics: Embracing the Myths, Traditions, Superstitions and Folk-lore of the Plant Kingdom* (S. Low, Marston, Searle & Rivington, New York, 1884).
65. Robisheaux, T., *The Last Witch of Langenburg: Murder in a German Village* (W.W. Norton, 2009).
66. Cunningham, S., *Cunningham's Encyclopaedia of Magical Herbs*, (2012)
67. Cockayne, T. O., *Leechdoms, Wortcunning and Starcraft* Vol. 1 (Cambridge University Press, 1864) 113.
68. Culpepper, N., *Culpepper's Complete Herbal and English Physician* (J. Greave & Son, Deansgate, Manchester, 1826).
69. Folkard, R., *Plant Lore, Legends, and Lyrics: Embracing the Myths, Traditions, Superstitions and Folk-lore of the Plant Kingdom* (S. Low, Marston, Searle & Rivington, New York, 1884).
70. Cockayne, T. O., *Leechdoms, Wortcunning and Starcraft* Vol. 1 (Cambridge University Press, 1864) 157.
71. Friend, J. N., *Demonology, Sympathetic Magic, and Witchcraft: A Study of Superstition as it Persists in Man and Affects Him in a Scientific Age* (C. Griffin, 1961).
72. Hyatt, H. M., *Hoodoo – Conjuration – Witchcraft – Rootwork* (Western Publishing Co., St. Louis, 1970).
73. Lecouteux, C., *Traditional Magic Spells for Protection and Healing* (Simon & Schuster, 2017).

74. Salmon, W., *Botanologia, the English Herbal, or History of Plants* (I. Dawks, London, 1710) 789.

75. Von Nettesheim, H. C., *The Philosophy of Natural Magic* (Jazzybee Verlag Jurgen Beck, 2014).

76. Hyatt, H. M., *Hoodoo – Conjuration – Witchcraft – Rootwork* (Western Publishing Co., St. Louis, 1970).

77. Della Porta, G., *Natural Magick* (John Wright, London, 1669).

78. Gerard, J., *The Herball or Generall Historie of Plantes* (John Norton, London, 1597).

79. Friend, J. N., *Demonology, Sympathetic Magic, and Witchcraft. A Study of Superstition as it Persists in Man and Affects Him in a Scientific Age* (C. Griffin, 1961).

80. Culpepper, N., *Culpepper's Complete Herbal and English Physician* (J. Greave & Son, Deansgate, Manchester, 1826).

81. Shakespeare, W, *Hamlet, Act IV, Scene 5* (Maynard, Merrill & Co., 1882) 126.

82. Langham, W., *The Garden of Health* (London, 1579) 483.

83. Cockayne, T. O., *Leechdoms, Wortcunning and Starcraft* Vol. 1 (Cambridge University Press, 1864)

84. Kochilas, D., *Ikaria* (Rodale Books, 2014).

85. Cockayne, T. O., *Leechdoms, Wortcunning and Starcraft* Vol. 1 (Cambridge University Press, 1864) 313

86. Lecouteux, C., *Traditional Magic Spells for Protection and Healing* (Simon & Schuster, 2017).

87. Folkard, R., *Plant Lore, Legends, and Lyrics: Embracing the Myths, Traditions, Superstitions and Folk-lore of the Plant Kingdom* (S. Low, Marston, Searle & Rivington, New York, 1884).

88. Northcote, R., *The Book of Herbs* (John Lane, London & New York, 1903).

89. Lesley, G., *Green Magic: Flowers, Plants and Herbs in Lore and Legend* (Viking Press, New York, 1977).

90. Kane, A., *Herbal Magic,* (Warfleet Press, 2021) 154.

91. Hyatt, H. M., *Hoodoo – Conjuration - Witchcraft – Rootwork* (Western Publishing Co., St. Louis, 1970) 2233.

92. Boswell, J., (ed.), *English Botany, or Coloured Figures of British Plants* (George Bell & Sons, London, 1878).

93. Ibid., 62.

94. Harvey, J., Daniel, Henry, *A Scientific Gardener of the Fourteenth Century*, Garden History, Vol. 15, No. 2, (1987) 81–93.

95. Folkard, R., *Plant Lore, Legends, and Lyrics: Embracing the Myths, Traditions, Superstitions and Folk-lore of the Plant Kingdom* (S. Low, Marston, Searle & Rivington, New York, 1884) 588.

96. Newcomb, W., *Newcomb's Midland counties' almanac and rural hand-book* (William Newcomb, London 1866).

97. Osborn, A. J., *Poison Hunting Strategies* (University of Nebraska, 2004).

98. Wexler, P. (ed.), *Toxicology in Antiquity*. Second Edition, (Elsevier, London & New York, 2019) 435.

99. Hill, J., *A History of the Materia Medica* Vol. 2 (Longman, London, 1751).

100. Bradley, R., *Dictionaire oeconomique: or The Family Dictionary* (D. Midwinter, London, 1725).

101. Pechey, J., *The Compleat Herbal of Physical Plants* (Henry Bonwicke, London, 1694).

102. Thomson, A., *The London Dispensatory* (Longman, Hurst, Rees, Orme & Brown, London, 1815).
103. Wright, P. (ed.), *The Poems of John Keats* (Wordsworth Editions Ltd, Hertfordshire, 1994).
104. Curie, P. H., *Domestic Homoeopathy* (Jesper Harding, Philadelphia, 1839).
105. Walafrid, S., *On the Cultivation of Gardens. A Ninth Century Gardening Book* (Ithuriel's Spear, San Francisco, 2009) 71.
106. British Newspaper Archive *Bath Chronicle and Weekly Gazette* (29 January 1767).
107. Scarborough, J., 'Ancient Medicinal Use of Aristolochia: Birthwort's Tradition and Toxicity', *Pharmacy in History*, Vol. 53, No. 1 (2011).
108. Gerard, J., *The Herball or Generall Historie of Plantes* (John Norton, London, 1597).
109. Burnett, G., Burnett, M. A. (ed.), *An Encyclopaedia of Useful and Ornamental Plants* (George Willis, London, 1852).
110. Northcote, R., *The Book of Herbs* (John Lane, London & New York, 1903).
111. Ellis, D., *Medicinal Herbs and Poisonous Plants* (Blackie & Son Limited, London, 1918) 31.
112. Fernie, W. T., *Herbal Simples* (John Wright & Co., Bristol, 1897).
113. Coles, W., *Adam in Eden, or Natures Paradise* (J. Streater, London, 1657) 575.
114. Fernie, W. T., *Herbal Simples* (John Wright & Co., Bristol, 1897).
115. Culpepper, N., *Culpepper's Complete Herbal and English Physician* (J. Greave & Son, Deansgate, Manchester, 1826).
116. Small, E., *North American Cornucopia* (2013).
117. Richards, M, *Hadrian's Wall Path, National Trail: Described West-East and east to West*, (Cicerone Press, 2020)
118. Fernie, W. T., *Herbal Simples* (John Wright & Co., Bristol, 1897).
119. Von Bingen, Hildegard & P. Throop (illus), *Hildegard von Bingen's Physica* (Healing Arts Press, Rochester, 1998) 43.
120. *Objections to the Treasury Minute, Legalising the Sale of Mixtures of Chicory and Coffee* (House of Lords, London, 1853) 6.
121. Gerard, J., *The Herball or Generall Historie of Plantes* (John Norton, London, 1597).
122. Culpepper, N., *Culpepper's Complete Herbal and English Physician* (J. Greave & Son, Deansgate, Manchester, 1826).
123. British Newspaper Archive *Derby Mercury* (28 June 1739).
124. Gerard, J., *The Herball or Generall Historie of Plantes* (John Norton, London, 1597).
125. *Caledonian Mercury* (13 August 1730).
126. Culpepper, N., *Culpepper's Complete Herbal and English Physician* (J. Greave & Son, Deansgate, Manchester, 1826) 38.
127. Dioscorides, P., *De Materia Medica* (IBIDIS Press, South Africa, 2000) 523.
128. Diederichsen, A., *Coriander* (International Plant Genetic Resources institute, Germany, 1996) 23.
129. Blackwell, E., *A Curious Herbal* Vol. 1 (John Norse, London, 1739.
130. Gerard, J., *The Herball or Generall Historie of Plantes* (John Norton, London, 1597).
131. Parkinson, J., *Paradisi in sole paradisus terrestris,* (Methuen & Co, 1904).
132. Von Bingen, Hildegard & P. Throop (illus), *Hildegard von Bingen's Physica* (Healing Arts Press, Rochester, 1998. 41.
133. Brueggermann, W., *Isiah 1–39* (Presbyterian Publishing Corporation, Westminster John Knox Press, Louisville & London, 1998) 229
134. Pereira, J., *The Elements of Materia Medica and Therapeutics* Vol. 2 part 2 (Longman, London, 1857) 167.

135. Parkinson, J., *Theatrum Botanicum* (The Cotes, London, 1640).
136. *Birmingham Medical Review* January–June Vol. 25 (J. & A. Churchill, London & Birmingham, 1889).
137. Culpepper, N., *Culpepper's Complete Herbal and English Physician* (J. Greave & Son, Deansgate, Manchester, 1826) 56.
138. *The Homeopathic Recorder* Vol. IV, (Boericke & Tafel, Philadelphia, 1889).
139. Von Bingen, Hildegard & P. Throop (illus), *Hildegard von Bingen's Physica* (Healing Arts Press, Rochester, 1998) 39–40.
140. Folkard, R., *Plant Lore, Legends, and Lyrics: Embracing the Myths, Traditions, Superstitions and Folk-lore of the Plant Kingdom* (S. Low, Marston, Searle & Rivington, New York, 1884) 349.
141. Bryan, C. P., *The Papyrus Ebers*, translated from the German (1930).
142. Shou-zhong, Y., *A Translation of the Shen Nong Ben Cao Jing* (Blue Poppy Press, 1998).
143. Parkinson, J., *Theatrum Botanicum* (The Cotes, London, 1640) 215.
144. Macht, D., *John Hopkins Medical Journal* Vol. 24 (John Hopkins Press, 1981).
145. Shakespeare, W., Delius, N., Symmons, C. (eds), *The Complete Works of William Shakespeare* (Baumgartner, Leipzig, 1864).
146. Andrew, T., *A Cyclopedia of Domestic Medicine and Surgery, etc* (Blackie & Son, Glasgow, 1842) 258.
147. Dioscorides, P., *De Materia Medica* (IBIDIS Press, South Africa, 2000) 29.
148. Fernie, W. T., *Herbal Simples* (John Wright & Co., Bristol, 1897).
149. *The Canon of Medicine* (AMS Press, New York, 1973).
150. Northcote, R., *The Book of Herbs* (John Lane, London & New York, 1903).
151. Dioscorides, P., *De Materia Medica* (IBIDIS Press, South Africa, 2000) 28.
152. Northcote, R., *The Book of Herbs* (John Lane, London & New York, 1903).
153. Pereira, J., *The Elements of Materia Medica and Therapeutics* Vol. 2, part 2 (Longman, London, 1857) 931.
154. Von Bingen, Hildegard & P. Throop (illus), *Hildegard von Bingen's Physica* (Healing Arts Press, Rochester, 1998) 22.
155. Andrew, T., *A Cyclopedia of Domestic Medicine and Surgery, etc* (Blackie & Son, Glasgow, 1842) 319.
156. Dioscorides, P., *De Materia Medica* (IBIDIS Press, South Africa, 2000) 503.
157. Green, Thomas, *The Universal Herbal* (Henry Fisher, Liverpool, 1820) 39.
158. Green, M. H., *The Trotula, An English Translation of the Medieval compendium of Women's Medicine* (University of Pennsylvania Press, 2002) 84.
159. Short, T., *Medicina Britannica* (R. Manby & H. Shute Cox, London, 1746).
160. Northcote, R., *The Book of Herbs* (John Lane, London & New York, 1903).
161. Dioscorides, P., *De Materia Medica* (IBIDIS Press, South Africa, 2000) 715.
162. Bryan, C. P., *The Papyrus Ebers*, translated from the German (1930).
163. Jones, W. H. S. (trans), Pliny, *Natural History, VII Books 24–27* (Harvard University Press, London, 1966) 357.
164. Dioscorides, P., *De Materia Medica* (IBIDIS Press, South Africa, 2000) 411.
165. Gerard, J., *The Herball or Generall Historie of Plantes* (John Norton, London, 1597).
166. Culpepper, N., *Culpepper's Complete Herbal and English Physician* (J. Greave & Son, Deansgate, Manchester, 1826) 106.
167. Wheeler, K., *A Natural History of Nettles*, (Trafford, Canada, 2007).
168. Green, M. H., *The Trotula, An English Translation of the Medieval Compendium of Women's Medicine.* (University of Pennsylvania Press, 2002) 109.

169. Rohde, E., *The Old English Herbals,* (Longmans, London, 1922).
170. Chaucer, Geoffrey, *The Miller's Prologue and Tale* (Cambridge University Press, Cambridge, 2016) 65.
171. Dioscorides, P., *De Materia Medica* (IBIDIS Press, South Africa, 2000).
172. Walafrid, S., *On the Cultivation of Gardens. A Ninth Century Gardening Book* (Ithuriel's Spear, San Francisco, 2009) 67.
173. Ibid.
174. Kochilas, D., *Ikaria* (Rodale Books, 2014) 54.
175. Pliny, *Natural History Vol. 7* (Harvard University Press, 1966).
176. Blackwell, E., *A Curious Herbal* Vol. 1 (John Norse, London, 1739).
177. Rawcliffe, C., 'Delectable Sightes and Fragrant Smelles': Gardens and Health in Late Medieval and Early Modern England, *Garden History* Vol. 36, No. 1 (2008).
178. Gerard, J. *The Herball or Generall Historie of Plantes* (John Norton, London, 1597).
179. Walafrid, S., *On the Cultivation of Gardens. A Ninth Century Gardening Book* (Ithuriel's Spear, San Francisco, 2009).
180. Fard, M. A., Shojaii, A., *Efficiency of Iranian Traditional Medicine in the Treatment of Epilepsy*, BioMed Research International (2013).
181. Kochilas, D., *Ikaria* (Rodale Books, 2014) 55.
182. Malim, C. T., *Practical Observations on the Properties of Garden Sage, as a Medicinal Agent,* (T. Bull, London, 1844).
183. Tildesley, N. T. et al., Salvia Lavandulaefolia (Spanish Sage) Enhances Memory in Healthy Young Volunteers, Pharmacology Biochemistry and Behaviour Vol. 75, Issue 3 (June (2003).
184. *The Diary of Samuel Pepys, Complete 1664* (Good Press, 2019).
185. Pereira, J, *The Elements of Materia Medica and Therapeutics* Vol 2 part 2 (Longman, London, 1857).
186. Dioscorides, P., *De Materia Medica* (IBIDIS Press, South Africa, 2000) 102.
187. Von Bingen, Hildegard & P. Throop (illus), *Hildegard von Bingen's Physica* (Healing Arts Press, Rochester, 1998).
188. Culpepper, N., *Culpepper's Complete Herbal and English Physician* (J. Greave & Son, Deansgate, Manchester, 1826) 155.
189. Shoemaker, J. V., *A Treatise on Materia Medica, Pharmacology, and Therapeutics* Vol. 2 (F. A. Davis, Philadelphia & London, 1891) 899.
190. Gerard, J., *The Herball or Generall Historie of Plantes* (John Norton, London, 1597).
191. Kochilas, D., *Ikaria* (Rodale Books, 2014) 55.
192. Evelyn, J., *Acetaria. A Discourse of Sallets* (Women's Auxiliary, Brooklyn, 1937).
193. Parkinson, J., *Paradisi in sole paradisus terrestri,* (Methuen & Co, 1904) 500.
194. Lemery, M. L., *Treatise of all Sorts of Food* (T. Osborne, London, 1745).
195. Short, T., *Medicina Britannica* (R. Manby & H. Shute Cox, London, 1746).
196. King, H., *The Disease of Virgins: Green Sickness, Chlorosis, and the Problems of Puberty* (Routledge, London, 2004).
197. Fernie, W. T., *Herbal Simples* (John Wright & Co., Bristol, 1897).
198. Walafrid, S., *On the Cultivation of Gardens. A Ninth Century Gardening Book* (Ithuriel's Spear, San Francisco, 2009).
199. Mahomoodally, M. F., *Traditional Medicines in Africa: An Appraisal of Ten Potent African Medicinal Plants* (Hindawi, 2013), www.hindawi.com/journals/ecam/2013/617459/ (accessed 12 March, 2021).
200. Riley, K. F., *Whispers in the Pines. The Secrets of Colliers Mills* (Cloonfad Press, New Jersey, 2005).

201. Cockayne, T.O., *Leechdoms, Wortcunning and Starcraft* Vol. 1 (Cambridge University Press, 1864) 197.

Chapter 3
1. Thoreau, H. D., The *Man Himself* (Musaicum Books, 2017).
2. Harvey, J, Daniel, Henry, *A Scientific Gardener of the Fourteenth Century*, Garden History, Vol .15 No. 2 (1987).
3. Pegge, S. (ed.), *Forme of Cury: A Roll of Ancient English Cookery. Compiled, about A.D. 1390, by the Master-Cooks of King RICHARD II* (1780), www.gutenberg.org/cache/epub/8102/pg8102.html (accessed 24 February 2021).
4. Ibid.
5. Spearing, A. C., *Readings in Medieval Poetry* (Cambridge University Press, 1989) 223.
6. Pegge, S. (ed.), *Forme of Cury: A Roll of Ancient English Cookery. Compiled, about A.D. 1390, by the Master-Cooks of King RICHARD II* (1780), www.gutenberg.org/cache/epub/8102/pg8102.html (accessed 24 February 2021).
7. Morris, R. (ed.), *Liber Cure Cocorum* (A. Asher & Co., Berlin, 1862).
8. Mollard, J., *The Art of Cookery Made Easy and Refined* (J. Nunn, London, 1808).
9. Anthonio, H. O., Isoun, M., *Nigerian Cookbook* (Macmillan, Hong Kong, 2009).
10. Prescott, J. (trans) *Le Viandier de Taillevent* (Alfarhaugr Publishing Society, Oregon, 1989), www.telusplanet.net/public/prescotj/data/viandier/viandier4.html (accessed 20 February 2021).
11. Pegge, S. (ed.), *Forme of Cury: A Roll of Ancient English Cookery. Compiled, about A.D. 1390, by the Master-Cooks of King RICHARD II* (1780), www.gutenberg.org/cache/epub/8102/pg8102.html (accessed 24 February 2021).
12. Gerard, J., *The Herball or Generall Historie of Plantes* (John Norton, London, 1597).
13. Ibid.
14. Murrell, J., *A New Booke of Cookerie* (London, 1615).
15. Molokhovets, E., Toomre, J. (trans), *Classic Russian Cooking. A Gift to Young Housewives* (Indiana University Press, Bloomington, 1992).
16. Acton, E., *Modern Cookery in all its Branches* (Lea & Blanchard, Philadelphia & London, 1845) 239.
17. Lecourt, H, *La Cuisine Chinoise* (Albert Nachbaur, Peking, 1925).
18. Cox, N., Dannehl, K., 'Valencia almond – Vermilion', in *Dictionary of Traded Goods and Commodities 1550–1820* (Wolverhampton, 2007), *British History Online*, www.british-history.ac.uk/no-series/traded-goods-dictionary/1550-1820/valencia-almond-vermilion (accessed 13 February 2021)
19. Bradley, R., *The Country Housewife and Lady's Director* (D. Browne, London, 1736) 16.
20. Dalrymple, G., *The Practice of Modern Cookery; Adapted to Families of Distinction, as Well as to Those of the Middling Ranks of Life* (Edinburgh, 1781) 46.
21. Kay, E., *Cooking up History: Chefs of the Past* (Prospect Books, London, 2017).
22. Senn, C. H., *The Book of Sauces* (Applewood Books, Massachusetts, 1915) 55.
23. Glasse, H., *The Complete Confectioner* (West & Hughes, London, 1800) 336.
24. *Ein Büch von Güter Speise* (Stuttgart, 1844) 17.
25. Muusers, C. (trans), *Wel ende edelike spijse* (Good and noble food), www.coquinaria.nl/kooktekst/Edelikespijse0.htm (accessed 6 May, 2021).

26. Austin, T., (ed.) Two fifteenth-century cookery-books: Harleian MS. 279 (ab. 1430), & Harleian MS. 4016 (ab. 1450), with extracts from Ashmole MS. 1439, Laud MS. 553, & Douce MS. 55. Fifteenth-century cookery book. 1. Harleian MS. 279, ab. 1420 (Oxford University Press, London, 1964)

27. *Kitab al-Tabeekh fi 'l-Maghrib wa 'l-Andalus fi 'Asr al-Muwahhidin* (The Cookbook of al-Maghrib and Andalusia in the era of the Almohads), http://daviddfriedman. com/Medieval/Cookbooks/Andalusian/andalusian7.htm#Heading360 (accessed 13 May, 2021).

28. De Monmarché, G. (trans), *Le Recueil de Riom*, www.erminespot.com/wp-content/uploads/2009/01/le-recueil-de-riom.pdf (accessed 13 May, 2021).

29. Jordan, P., *Field Guide to Edible Mushrooms* (Bloomsbury, 2015).

30. W.M., *The Compleat Cook* (Nath Brook, London, 1658).

31. Forest, M. (trans), *Koge Bog* (Cook book) (Salomone Sartorio, Copenhagen, 1616), www.forest.gen.nz/Medieval/articles/cooking/1616.html (accessed 20 May 2021).

32. British Newspaper Archive, *Perthshire Advertiser* (8 October 1993).

33. *Sengoku Daimyo*, 2019. https://sengokudaimyo.com/rm-ch12 (accessed 22 May 2021).

34. A. W.. *A Book of Cookrye Very Necessary for all Such as Delight Therin* (Edward Allde, London, 1591).

35. Copley, E., *The Cook's Complete Guide on the Principles of Frugality, Comfort and Elegance* (George Virtue, London, 1810) 73.

36. Plimmer, V., *Food Values in Wartime* (Longmans, Green & Co., London, New York, and Toronto, 1941).

37. Murrell, J., *A New Book of Cookerie* (London, 1615).

38. W.M., *The Compleat Cook* (Nath Brook, London, 1658).

39. Kuper, J., *The Anthropologist's Cookbook* (Routledge, London & New York, 2009) 24.

40. Chatto, J., Martin, W. L., *A Kitchen in Corfu* (New Amsterdam Books, New York, 1988) 36,

41. Weiss Adamson, M. (ed.), *Food in the Middle Ages* (Taylor & Francis, Oxford, 1995).

42. Stopp, H. (ed.), *The Cookbook by Sabina Welserin* (University of Heidelberg, Germany, 1980).

43. Friedman, D. (trans), *The Cookbook of Sabrina Welserin*, www.daviddfriedman. com/Medieval/Cookbooks/Sabrina_Welserin.html, (accessed 20 May, 2021).

44. Cook, E. (trans), *Maistre Chiquart, Du fait de cuisine*, www.daviddfriedman. com/Medieval/Cookbooks/Du_Fait_de_Cuisine/Du_fait_de_Cuisine.html (accessed 14 June, 2021).

45. British Newspaper Archive *Burnley Express* (18 April 1936).

46. Kitchiner, William, *The Cook's Oracle* (Robert Cadell, Edinburgh, 1845) 204.

47. Abu Muhammad al-Muthaffar ibn Nasr ibn Sayyār al-Warrāq, Nawal Nasrallah (trans), *Annals of the Caliphs' Kitchens* (Brill, The Netherlands, 2007).

48. Markham, G., *The English Huswife* (Hannah Sawbridge, London, 1615).

49. *Sengoku Daimyo*, 2019 https://sengokudaimyo.com/rm-ch12 (accessed, 22, May 2021).

50. Walton, I., *The Complete Angler* (C. & C. Whittingham, London, 1826) 261.

51. Pegge, S. (ed.), *Forme of Cury: A Roll of Ancient English Cookery. Compiled, about A.D. 1390, by the Master-Cooks of King RICHARD II* (1780), www.gutenberg.org/cache/epub/8102/pg8102.html (accessed 24 February 2021).

52. Du Libre B, From *Due Libri di Cucina*, www.daviddfriedman.com/Medieval/Cookbooks/Due_Libre_B/Due_Libre_B.pdf (accessed, 15, June, 2021).

53. Tusser, T., *Five Hundred Pointes of Good Husbandrie* (Trubner & Co, London, 1878).

54. *Libre del Coch, 1529*, www.florilegium.org/files/FOOD-MANUSCRIPTS/Guisados1-art.html (accessed 15 June 2021).

55. Ibid.

56. Power, E. (ed), *The Goodman of Paris. A Treatise on Moral and Domestic Economy by a Citizen of Paris* (Boydell Press, Woodbridge, 2006) 180.

57. Larson, H., *An Old Icelandic Medical Miscellany* (Oslo, 1931).

58. Hieatt, C. B, Grewe, R. (ed), *Libellus de Arte Coquinaria. An Early Northern Cookery Book* (Arizona Centre for Medieval Renaissance Studies, 2001) 73.

59. Strybel, M., Strybel, R., *Polish Heritage Cookery* (Hippocrene Books, New York, 1993).

60. Dembinska, M., *Food and Drink in Medieval Poland. Rediscovering a Cuisine of the Past* (University of Pennsylvania Press, 1999) 93.

61. Chen, S. J. S., *The Way of Eating* (Berkshire Publishing Group, 2019).

62. Pegge, S. (ed.), *Forme of Cury: A Roll of Ancient English Cookery. Compiled, about A.D. 1390, by the Master-Cooks of King RICHARD II* (1780), www.gutenberg.org/cache/epub/8102/pg8102.html (accessed 24 February 2021).

63. Mackenzie, Colin, *Mackenzie's Five Thousand Receipts, in all Useful and Domestic Arts* (James Kay Jun & Co., Philadelphia & John I. Kay & Co., Pittsburgh, 1831).

64. Kovacs, B. (trans), *The Prince of Transylvania's Court Master Chef.* Glenn Gorsuch (ed.), *The Prince of Transylvania's Court Cookbook, from the 16th Century. The Science of Cooking*, www.medievalcookery.com/etexts/transylvania-v2.pdf (accessed 27 April 2021).

65. al-Muẓaffar ibn Naṣr Ibn Sayyār al-Warrāq, Kaj Öhrnberg, Saḥbān Murūwah, *Annals of the Caliph's Kitchens* (Brill, 2007, Netherlands) 440.

66. Rooibos and Buchu lamb shanks, https://static1.squarespace.com/static/564312e0e4b02d0ff72509f3/t/5e7da228b4d27021652c94df/1585292816689/Rooibos+lamb+shank (accessed, 20 April 2021).

67. Gate, W., *An Aztec Herbal,* (Dover Publications, New York, 2000).

68. De Oliveira Marques, A. H. R. & S. Wyatt, *Daily Life in Portugal in the Late Middle Ages* (University of Wisconsin Press, Madison, WI, 1971).

69. Gomes, F. (trans), *A Treatise of Portuguese Cuisine from the 15th Century* (2007), www.medievalcookery.com/notes/tratado.html (accessed 1 May 2021).

70. Titley, N. M. (trans), *The Ni'matnama Manuscript of the Sultans of Mandu* (Routledge, London, 2004) 10,

71. Christies, H., *Banquets of the Nations; Eighty-six Dinners Characteristic and Typical Each of its Own Country* (J. & J. Gray, Edinburgh, 1911) 387.

72. Pegge, S. (ed.), *Forme of Cury: A Roll of Ancient English Cookery. Compiled, about A.D. 1390, by the Master-Cooks of King RICHARD II* (1780), www.gutenberg.org/cache/epub/8102/pg8102.html (accessed 24 February 2021).

73. Black, F., *The Art of Giving* (Fowler Wright Books, Leominster, 1990) 167.

74. Kovacs, B. (trans), *The Prince of Transylvania's Court Master Chef.* Glenn Gorsuch (ed.), *The Prince of Transylvania's Court Cookbook, from the 16th Century. The Science of Cooking*, www.medievalcookery.com/etexts/transylvania-v2.pdf (accessed 27 April 2021).

75. Perry, C. (trans), *An Anonymous Andalusian Cookbook of the 13th Century*, http://daviddfriedman.com/Medieval/Cookbooks/Andalusian/andalusian_contents.htm/ (accessed 24 April 2021)

76. Nott, J., *The Cooks and Confectioners Dictionary* (C. Rivington, London, 1723).

77. Moore, R., *The Artizan's Guide* (John Lovell, Montreal, 1878) 93.

78. Cox, N, Dannehl, K., 'Caracca nut – Carduus water', in *Dictionary of Traded Goods and Commodities 1550–1820* (Wolverhampton, 2007), *British History Online*, www.british-history.ac.uk/no-series/traded-goods-dictionary/1550-1820/caracca-nut-carduus-water (accessed 12 February 2021).

79. Sanderson, J. M., *The Complete Cook* (W.A. Leary, Philadelphia, 1850) 45.

80. Gerard, J., *The Herball or Generall Historie of Plantes* (John Norton, London, 1597).

81. Plat, Hugh, *Delightes for Ladies, to Adorne Their Persons* (Humfrey Lownes, London, 1609).

82. Anon, *A Queens Delight* (1671).

83. Nutt, F., *The Complete Confectioner* (Richard Scott, London, 1807) 33.

84. Jarrin, W., *The Italian Confectioner*, (William H. Ainsworth, London, 1827).

85. Lee, N., *The American Family Cook Book*, (Higgins, Bradley & Dayton, Boston, 1858) 284.

86. De la Cruz, M. & William Gates (ed.), *An Aztec Herbal. The Classic Codex of 1552* (Dover Publications, New York, NY, 2000) 37.

87. McNeill, F. M., *The Scots Kitchen*, (Mercat Press, Edinburgh) 233

88. Pegge, S. (ed.), *Forme of Cury: A Roll of Ancient English Cookery. Compiled, about A.D. 1390, by the Master-Cooks of King RICHARD II* (1780), www.gutenberg.org/cache/epub/8102/pg8102.html (accessed 24 February 2021).

89. Digbie K., *The Closet of the Eminently Learned Sir Kenelme Digbie Knight, Opened* (1669).

90. Roberts, W. H., *The British Wine-maker and Domestic Brewer* (A. & C. Black, Edinburgh, 1849) 241.

91. Hannah, G., *The Complete Confectioner, Or Housekeeper's Guide* (J. W. Meyers, 1800).

92. Dioscorides, P., *De Materia Medica* (IBIDIS Press, South Africa, 2000) 769.

93. Bamforth, C. W, Ward, R. E., *The Oxford Handbook of Food Fermentations* (Oxford University Press, Oxford, 2014).

94. Ricket E., Thomas, C., *The Gentleman's Table Guide* (Agent-H Born, London, 1871).

95. *Cassell's Dictionary of Cookery* (Cassell, Petter, Galpin & Co., London, Paris, and New York, 1883) 815–16.

Bibliography

Publications

A Cyclopedia of Domestic Medicine and Surgery, etc. (Blackie & Son, Glasgow, 1842).

A History of Magic and Experimental Science Vol. 1 (Columbia University Press, New York & London, 1923).

A History of Magic and Experimental Science Vol. 1 (Columbia University Press, New York & London, 1923).

A. W.. *A Book of Cookrye Very Necessary for all Such as Delight Therin* (Edward Allde, London, 1591).

Abu Muhammad al-Muthaffar ibn Nasr ibn Sayyār al-Warrāq, Nawal Nasrallah (trans) *Annals of the Caliphs' Kitchens* (Brill, The Netherlands, 2007).

Acton, E., *Modern Cookery in all its Branches*, (Lea & Blanchard, Philadelphia & London, 1845).

al-Muẓaffar ibn Naṣr Ibn Sayyār al-Warrāq, Kaj Öhrnberg, Saḥbān Murūwah, *Annals of the Caliph's Kitchens* (Brill, The Netherlands, 2007).

Amherst, A., *A History of Gardening in England* (Bernard Quaritch, London, 1895).

Andrew, T., *A Cyclopedia of Domestic Medicine and Surgery, etc* (Blackie & Son, Glasgow, 1842).

Anon, *A Queens Delight*, (1671).

Anthonio, H. O. & M. Isou, *Nigerian Cookbook* (Macmillan, Hong Kong, 2009).

Atkinson, T., *Napier's History of Herbal Healing* (Creative Print & Design, Wales, 2003).

Austin, T., (ed.) Two fifteenth-century cookery-books: Harleian MS. 279 (ab. 1430), & Harleian MS. 4016 (ab. 1450), with extracts from Ashmole MS. 1439, Laud MS. 553, & Douce MS. 55. Fifteenth-century cookery book. 1. Harleian MS. 279, ab. 1420 (Oxford University Press, London, 1964)

Avicenna, *The Canon of Medicine* (AMS Press, New York, NY, 1973).

Bamforth, C. W. & R. E. Ward, *The Oxford Handbook of Food Fermentations* (Oxford University Press, Oxford, 2014).

Baynes, R. H. (ed.), *The Churchman's Shilling Magazine and Family Treasury* Vol. 16, (Houlston & Sons, London, 1874).

Bellshill Speaker, Saturday, 28 December 1901.

Birmingham Medical Review January–June Vol. 25 (J&A Churchill, London & Birmingham, 1889).

Black, F., *The Art of Giving* (Fowler Wright Books, Leominster, 1990).

Blackwell, E., *A Curious Herbal* Vol. 1 (John Norse, London, 1739).

Boswell, J. (ed.), *English Botany, or, Coloured Figures of British Plants.* (George Bell & Sons, London, 1878).

Bottéro, J., 'The Culinary Tablets at Yale', *Journal of the American Oriental Society*, Vol. 107, No. 1 (1987).

Bradley, R., *Dictionaire oeconomique: or The Family Dictionary.* (D. Midwinter, London, 1725).

Bradley, R., *The Country Housewife and Lady's Director* (D. Browne, London, 1736).

British Newspaper Archive *Belfast News-letter* (25 December 1905).

British Newspaper Archive *Bellshill Speaker* (28 December, 1901).

British Newspaper Archive *Edinburgh Evening News* (7 January 1884).

British Newspaper Archive *Edinburgh Evening News* (7 January 1884).

British Newspaper Archive *Lancashire Eve Post* (25 July 1957).

British Newspaper Archive *Lancashire Evening Post* (25 July 1957).

British Newspaper Archive *Lancashire Evening Post* (15 August 1933).

British Newspaper Archive *Lancashire Evening Post* (15 August 1933).

British Newspaper Archive *Nottingham Journal* (Thursday 23 October 1913).

British Newspaper Archive *Sheffield Daily Telegraph* (29 November 1855).

British Newspaper Archive *Sheffield Daily Telegraph* (29 November 1855).

British Newspaper Archive *Bath Chronicle and Weekly Gazette* (29 January 1767).

British Newspaper Archive *Bradford Observer* (25 February 1943).

British Newspaper Archive *Burnley Express* (18 April 1936).

British Newspaper Archive *Derby Mercury* (28 June 1739).

British Newspaper Archive *Edinburgh Evening News* (5 May 1939).

British Newspaper Archive, *Perthshire Advertiser* (8 October 1993).

Britten, W., *Art magic, or mundane, sub-mundane and super-mundane spiritism* (New York, 1876).

Britten, W. & E. Britten, *Art Magic, or Mundane, Sub-mundane and Super-mundane Spiritism: An English Translation of the Medieval Compendium of Women's Medicine* (University of Pennsylvania Press, PA, 2002).

Brooke, E., *Women Healers Through History* (Aeon Books, 2020)

Brown, P., *Botanical Drawing* (Search Press, 2017).

Brown, P. C., *Essex Witches* (The History Press, Brimscombe, 2014).

Brueggermann, W., *Isiah 1–39* (Presbyterian Publishing Corporation, Westminster John Knox Press, Louisville & London, 1998).

Bryan, C.P., *The Papyrus Ebers*, translated from the German (1930).

Burnett, G. & M. A. Burnett (eds). *An Encyclopaedia of Useful and Ornamental Plants* (George Willis, London, 1852)

Caledonian Mercury (13 August, 1730).

Cassell's Dictionary of Cookery (Cassell, Petter, Galpin & Co., London, Paris & New York, 1883).

Chatto, J. & Martin, W. L., *A Kitchen in Corfu* (New Amsterdam Books, New York, 1988).

Chaucer, Geoffrey, *The Canterbury Tales* (Oxford University Press, Oxford & New York, 2011).

Chaucer, Geoffrey, *The Miller's Prologue and Tale* (Cambridge University Press, Cambridge, 2016).

Chen, S. J. S., *The Way of Eating* (Berkshire Publishing Group, USA, 2019).

Christies, H., *Banquets of the Nations; Eighty-six Dinners Characteristic and Typical Each of its Own Country* (J. & J. Gray, Edinburgh, 1911).

Cockayne, T. O., *Leechdoms, Wortcunning and Starcraft* Vol. 1 (Cambridge University Press, Cambridge, 1864)

Coles, W., *Adam in Eden, or Natures Paradise* (J. Streater, London, 1657).

Copley, E., *The Cook's Complete Guide on the Principles of Frugality, Comfort and Elegance* (George Virtue, London, 1810).

Creese, M. R. C. & T. Creese, *Ladies in the Laboratory III* (The Scarecrow Press, Plymouth, 2010).

Culpeper, N, *Culpeper's Complete Herbal* (J. Gleve & Son, Manchester 1826).

Culpepper, N., *Culpepper's Complete Herbal and English Physician* (J. Greave & Son, Deansgate, Manchester, 1826).

Cunningham, S., *Cunningham's Encyclopaedia of Magical Herbs* (2012).

Curie, P. H, *Domestic Homoeopathy* (Jesper Harding, Philadelphia, 1839).

Curran, R., *A Bewitched Land. Ireland's Witches* (The O'Brien Press, Ireland, 2012).

Dalrymple, G., *The Practice of Modern Cookery; Adapted to Families of Distinction, as Well as to Those of the Middling Ranks of Life* (Edinburgh, 1781).

Da Silva, Z., *The Herb in History, Mysteries and Crafts* (Cambridge Scholars Publishing, Newcastle upon Tyne, 2017).

Davies, O., *Witchcraft, Magic and Culture, 1736–1951* (Manchester University Press, Manchester, 1999).

De la Cruz, M. & William Gates (ed.), *An Aztec Herbal. The Classic Codex of 1552* (Dover Publications, New York, NY, 2000).

De Oliveira Marques, A. H. R. & S. Wyatt, *Daily Life in Portugal in the Late Middle Ages* (University of Wisconsin Press, Madison, WI, 1971).

Delany, P., *Constantinus Africanus' 'De Coitu'*: A Translation, *The Chaucer Review*, Vol. 4, No. 1, (Penn State University Press, PA).

Della Porta, G., *Natural Magick* (John Wright, London, 1669).

Dembinska, M., *Food and Drink in Medieval Poland. Rediscovering a Cuisine of the Past* (University of Pennsylvania Press, PA, 1999).

Denham, Alison M., *Herbal Medicine in Nineteenth Century England: The Career of John Skelton* (University of York, Yorkshire, 2013).

Diederichsen, A., *Coriander* (International Plant Genetic Resources Institute, Germany, 1996).

Digbie K., *The Closet of the Eminently Learned Sir Kenelme Digbie Knight, Opened* (1669).

Dioscorides, P., *De Materia Medica* (IBIDIS Press, South Africa, 2000).

Dyer, T. F., *The Folklore of Plants* (Appleton & Co., New York, 1889).

Ebsworth, J., (ed.), *The Roxburghe Ballards* (Stephen Austin & Sons, Hertford, 1893).

Ein Büch von Güter Speise (Stuttgart, Germany, 1844).

Ellis, D., *Medicinal Herbs and Poisonous Plants* (Blackie & Son Limited, London, 1918).

Evelyn, J., *Acetaria. A Discourse of Sallets*, (Women's Auxiliary, Brooklyn, NY, 1937).

Fard, M. A. & A. Shojaii, 'Efficiency of Iranian Traditional Medicine in the Treatment of Epilepsy', *BioMed Research International* (2013).

Fernie, W. T., *Herbal Simples* (John Wright & Co., Bristol, 1897).

Folkard, R., *Plant Lore, Legends and Lyrics: Embracing the Myths, Traditions, Superstitions and Folk-lore of the Plant Kingdom* (S. Low, Marston, Searle & Rivington, New York, NY, 1884).

Forbes, T. R., *The Midwife and the Witch*, (AMS Press, New York, NY, 1982).

Foust, C., *Rhubarb: The Wonderous Drug* (Princeton University Press, NJ, 1992).

Friend, H., *Flowers and Flower Lore* (W. S. Sonnenschein, 1884).

Friend, J. N., *Demonology, Sympathetic Magic and Witchcraft. A Study of Superstition as it Persists in Man and Affects Him in a Scientific Age* (C. Griffin, London, 1961).

Furnivall, F. J., *Harrison's Description of England in Shakespeare's Youth* (The New Shakespeare Society, London, 1877).

Gamache. H, *The Magic of Herbs* (Health Research, 1972).

Gate, W., *An Aztec Herbal* (Dover Publications, New York, NY, 2000).

George, A., *A Banksia Album* (National Library of Australia, Canberra, ACT, 2011).

Gerard, J., *The Herball or Generall Historie of Plantes* (John Norton, London, 1597).

Gimassi, R., *Old World Witchcraft* (Weiser Books, San Francisco, CA, 2011).

Glasse, H., *The Complete Confectioner* (West & Hughes, London, 1800).

Green, M. H., *The Trotula, An English Translation of the Medieval compendium of Women's Medicine* (University of Pennsylvania Press, PA, 2002).

Greene, R., *Quip for an Upstart Courtier* (1592).

Grieve, Maud, *A Modern Herbal* Vol. 1, (Dover Publications, Mineola, NY, 1931).

Griggs, B., *Helpful Herbs for Health and Beauty* (Infinite Ideas, Kindle, 2008).

Hajar, R., 'The Air of History (Part II) Medicine in the Middle Ages', *History of Medicine* Vol. 13, issue 4 (2012).

Halsbury's Statutes of England Vol. 21 (Butterworths, London, 1970).

Hannah, G., *The Complete Confectioner, Or Housekeeper's Guide* (J. W. Meyers, 1800).

Hartland, E. S., *The Legend of Perseus* (D. Nutt, London, 1894).

Harvey, J. & Henry Daniel, 'A Scientific Gardener of the Fourteenth Century', *Garden History* Vol 15, No. 2 (1987).

Harvey, J. H., 'Garden Plants of Around 1525: The Fromond List', *Garden History* Vol. 17, No. 2 (1989).

Harvey, J. H., 'The Square Garden of Henry the Poet', *Garden History* Vol. 15, No. 1 (1987).

Hieatt, C. B. & R. Grewe (ed.), *Libellus de Arte Coquinaria: An Early Northern Cookery Book* (Arizona Centre for Medieval and Renaissance Studies, Tempe, AZ, 2001).

Hill, J., *A History of the Materia Medica* Vol. 2 (Longman, London, 1751).

Homer, R. Fagles & B. Know (eds) *The Odyssey* (Penguin Books, London, 2002).

Hunting, P., *The Worshipful Society of Apothecaries of London* (BMJ Publishing Group, London, 2004).

Hyatt, H. M., *Hoodoo – Conjuration – Witchcraft – Rootwork* (Western Publishing Co., St. Louis, MO, 1970).

Illes, J., *Pure Magic. A Complete Course in Spellcasting* (Weiser Books, San Francisco, CA, 2007).

Isely, D., *One Hundred and One Botanists* (Purdue University Press, West Lafayette, IN, 2002).

Jackson, Helen Hunt, *September* (1892).

Jalkson, L., *Ten Centuries of European Progress* (Sampson Low, Marston & Co. Ltd., London, 1893).

Jarrin, W., *The Italian Confectioner* (William H. Ainsworth, London, 1827).

Jonson, Ben, W. Gifford (ed.) *The Works of Ben Jonson with a Biographical Memoir* (George Routledge & Sons, London & New York, 1869).

Jordan, P., *Field Guide to Edible Mushrooms* (Bloomsbury, London, 2015).

Kane, A., *Herbal Magic,* (Warfleet Press, USA, 2021)

Kay, E., *Cooking up History: Chefs of the Past,* (Prospect Books, London, 2017).

Keene, D. J. & V. Harding, 'St. Pancras Soper Lane 145/30', in *Historical Gazetteer of London Before the Great Fire Cheapside; Parishes of All Hallows Honey Lane, St Martin Pomary, St Mary Le Bow, St Mary Colechurch and St Pancras Soper Lane* (London, 1987). *British History Online* www.british-history.ac.uk/no-series/london-gazetteer-pre-fire/pp766-767 (accessed 13 March 2021).

Kelley, T. M., *Clandestine Marriage. Botany and Romantic Culture* (Johns Hopkins University Press, Baltimore, MD, 2012).

Kieschnick, J., *The Eminent Monk. Buddhist Ideals in Medieval Chinese Hagiography* (Kuroda Institute, Hawaii, 1997).

King, H., *The Disease of Virgins: Green Sickness, Chlorosis and the Problems of Puberty* (Routledge, London, 2004).

King, S. & G. Timmins, *Making Sense of the Industrial Revolution English Economy and Society 1700–1850* (Manchester University Press, Manchester, 2001).

Kitchiner, William, *The Cook's Oracle* (Robert Cadell, Edinburgh, 1845).

Knight, C., *London* Vols 1–2, (Charles Knight & Co., London, 1841).

Kochilas, D., *Ikaria* (Rodale Books, Emmaus, PA, 2014)

Kuper, J., *The Anthropologist's Cookbook* (Routledge, London & New York, 2009).

Landsberg, S., *The Medieval Garden* (University of Toronto Press, Toronto, 2003).

Langham, W., *The Garden of Health* (London, 1579).

Larson, H., *An Old Icelandic Medical Miscellany* (Oslo, Norway, 1931).

Lecourt, H., *La Cuisine Chinoise* (Albert Nachbaur, Peking, 1925).

Lecouteux, C., *The High Magic of Talismans and Amulets, Tradition and Craft* (Simon & Schuster, London, 2014).

Lecouteux, C., *Traditional Magic Spells for Protection and Healing* (Simon & Schuster, London, 2017).

Lee, N., *The American Family Cook Book*, (Higgins, Bradley & Dayton, Boston, MA, 1858.)

Lees, E., *The Botanical Looker-out Among the Wild Flowers of the Fields, Woods and Mountains of England and Wales* (Hamilton, Adams & Co., 1851).

Lemery, M. L., *Treatise of all Sorts of Food* (T. Osborne, London, 1745).

Leong, E., '"Herbals She Peruseth": Reading Medicine in Early Modern England', *Renaissance Studies* Vol. 28, No. 4 (2014).

Lesley, G., *Green Magic: Flowers, Plants and Herbs in Lore and Legend* (Viking Press, New York, NY, 1977).

Levack, B. P., *Witchcraft in Scotland* (Garland Publishing Inc., New York & London, 1992).

Leyel, C. F., *Cinquefoil* (Faber & Faber, London, 1957).

Macht, D., *John Hopkins Medical Journal* Vol. 24 (John Hopkins Press, Baltimore, MD, 1981).

Mackenzie, Colin, *Mackenzie's Five Thousand Receipts, in all Useful and Domestic Arts* (James Kay Jun & Co., Philadelphia & John I. Kay & Co., Pittsburgh, 1831).

Madge, B., *Elizabeth Blackwell: The Forgotten Herbalist?* (Wiley Online Library, 2003).

Malim, C. T., *Practical Observations on the Properties of Garden Sage, as a Medicinal Agent* (T. Bull, London, 1844).

Markham, G., *The English Huswife* (Hannah Sawbridge, London, 1615).

Marland, H., *Medicine and Society in Wakefield and Huddersfield 1780–1870* (Cambridge University Press, Cambridge, 1987).

Mayhew, H., *London Labour and the London Poor* Vol. 1 (Griffin, Bohn & Co., 1861).

McNeill, F. M., *The Scots Kitchen* (Mercat Press, Edinburgh, 2004).

Minter, Sue, *The Apothecaries' Garden* (The History Press, Brimscombe, 2000).

Minter, Sue, *The Well-Connected Gardener: A Biography of Alicia Amherst* (The Book Guild Ltd, Kibworth, 2010).

Mollard, J., *The Art of Cookery Made Easy and Refined* (J. Nunn, London, 1808).

Molokhovets, E., J. Toomre, J (trans), *Classic Russian Cooking. A Gift to Young Housewives* (Indiana University Press, Bloomington, IN, 1992).

Monod, P. K., *Solomon's Secret Arts* (Yale University Press, New Haven & London, 2013) .

Moor, S., *The Publican's Friend, and Sure Guide to Do Well* (1812).

Moore, R., *The Artizan's Guide* (John Lovell, Montreal, 1878).

Morris, R. (ed.), *Liber Cure Cocorum* (A. Asher & Co., Berlin, 1862).

Murrell, J., *A New Booke of Cookerie* (London, 1615).

Murrey, T. J., *Salads and Sauces* (Frederick A. Stokes, New York, NY, 1884).

Newcomb, W., *Newcomb's Midland Counties' Almanac and Rural Hand-book* (William Newcomb, London, 1866).

North, M., J. Symonds (ed.) *Recollections of a Happy Life, Being the Autobiography of Marianne North* (Macmillan, New York, 1894).

Northcote, R., *The Book of Herbs* (John Lane, London & New York, 1903).

Notes and Queries Vol. 5, January–June (John Francis, London, 1876).

Nott, J., *The Cooks and Confectioners Dictionary* (C. Rivington, London, 1723).

Nutt, F., *The Complete Confectioner* (Richard Scott, London, 1807).

Objections to the Treasury Minute, legalising the sale of mixtures of Chicory and Coffee (House of Lords, London, 1853).

Olav, T., *Nicholas Culpeper: English Physician and Astrologer* (Palgrave Macmillan, London, 1992).

Osborn, A. J, *Poison Hunting Strategies*, (University of Nebraska Press, Lincoln, NE, 2004).

Parkinson, A., *Nature's Alchemist* (Francis Lincoln Ltd, London, 2007).

Parkinson, J., *A Garden of all Sorts of Pleasant Flowers* (Humfrey Lownes & Robert Young, London, 1629).

Parkinson, J., *Paradisi in sole paradisus terrestris* (Methuen & Co, London, 1904).

Parkinson, J., *Theatrum Botanicum* (The Cotes, London, 1640).

Parkinson, S., *A Journal of a Voyage to the South Seas, in His Majesty's Ship The Endeavour* (London, 1773).

Payne, R. (trans), *Hortulus. De Cultura hortulorum* (Hunt Botanical Library, Pittsburgh, PA, 1966).

Pechey, J., *The Compleat Herbal of Physical Plants* (Henry Bonwicke, London, 1694).

Pegge, S., *Curialia \Miscellanea* (J. Nichols, Son & Bentley, London, 1818).

Pennick, N., *Operative Witchcraft* (Destiny Books, Rochester, VT, 2019).

Pereira, J., *The Elements of Materia Medica and Therapeutics* Vol. 2, Part 2 (Longman, London, 1857).

Pett, D. E. & A. Hodge, *The Cornwall Gardens Guide* (Alison Hodge, 2006).

Plat, Hugh, *Delightes for Ladies, to Adorne Their Persons.* (Humfrey Lownes, London, 1609).

Plat, Hugh, *The Garden of Eden* (1653).

Plimmer, V., *Food Values in Wartime* (Longmans, Green & Co., London, New York and Toronto, 1941).

Pliny, W. H. S Jones (trans), *Natural History*, Vol. VII, Books 24–27 (Harvard University Press, London, 1966).

Powell, R., 'The Magical Flower Used in Invisibility Ointments and Flying Powders', *Sydney Morning Herald* (Sydney, 2021).

Power, E. (ed.), *The Goodman of Paris. A Treatise on Moral and Domestic Economy by a Citizen of Paris* (Boydell Press, Woodbridge, 2006).

Public Opinion Vol. 20 (London, 1871).

Raven, C. E., *John Ray Naturalist: His Life and Works* (Cambridge University Press, Cambridge, London, New York, Melbourne, New Rochelle & Sydney, 1950).

Rawcliffe, C., 'Delectable Sightes and Fragrant Smelles: Gardens and Health in Late Medieval and Early Modern England'. *Garden History* Vol. 36, No. 1 (2008).

Rhode, E., *The Old English Herbals* (Minerva Press, London, 1974).

Richards, M., *Hadrian's Wall Path, National Trail: Described West–East and East–West* (Cicerone Press, Kendal, 2020).

Ricket E. & C. Thomas, *The Gentleman's Table Guide* (Agent-H Born, London, 1871).

Riley, K. F., *Whispers in the Pines. The Secrets of Colliers Mills* (Cloonfad Press, Cassville, NJ, 2005).

Roberts, W. H., *The British Wine-maker and Domestic Brewer* (A. & C. Black, Edinburgh, 1849).

Robisheaux, T., *The Last Witch of Langenburg: Murder in a German Village* (W. W. Norton & Co, New York, NY, 2009).

Rohde, E., *The Old English Herbals*, (Longmans, London, 1922).

Rousseau, G., *The Notorious Sir John Hill* (Lehigh University Press, Bethlehem, PA, 2012).

Rowland B., *Medieval Guide to Women's Health* (Kent University Press, Kent, OH, 1981).

Salmon, W. *Botanologia, the English Herbal, or History of Plants* (I. Dawks, London, 1710).

Sanderson, J. M., *The Complete Cook* (W. A. Leary, Philadelphia, PA, 1850).

Scarborough, J., 'Ancient Medicinal Use of Aristolochia: Birthwort's Tradition and Toxicity', *Pharmacy in History*, Vol. 53, No. 1 (2011).

Schwemer, D., G. van Buylaere, M. Luukko & T. Abusch, *Corpus of Mesopotamian Anti-Witchcraft Rituals* Vol. 3 (Brill, Leiden & Boston, 2020).

Sellar, A. M., *Bede's Ecclesiastical History of England, A Revised Translation* (George Bell & Sons, London, 1907).

Shakespeare, W., N. Delius & C. Symmons (eds), *The Complete Works of William Shakespeare*, (Baumgartner, Leipzig, 1864).

Shakespeare, W., *Hamlet, Act IV, Scene 5* (Maynard, Merrill & Co., 1882).

Shakespeare, W., *Romeo and Juliet, Act V, Scene 1* (Stanley Thornes, UK, 2014).

Shakespeare, W., *The Oxford Shakespeare: Richard II* (Oxford University Press, Oxford, 2011).

Sheppard, Edgar, Memorials of St. James's Palace Vol. 1 (Longmans, Green & Co., London, 1894).

Sheppard, F. H. (ed.), 'Covent Garden Market', *Survey of London* Vol. 36 (Covent Garden, London, 1970).

Shoemaker, J. V., *A Treatise on Materia Medica, Pharmacology, and Therapeutics* Vol. 2 (F. A. Davis, Philadelphia & London, 1891).

Short, T., *Medicina Britannica* (R. Manby & H. Shute Cox, London, 1746).

Shou-zhong, Y., *A Translation of the Shen Nong Ben Cao Jing* (Blue Poppy Press, North Devon, 1998).

Sibly, E., *A Key to Physic, and the Occult Sciences* (London, 1795).

Simoons, F. J., *Plants of Life, Plants of Death*, (University of Wisconsin Press, Madison, WI, 1998).

Sloane, H., *An Account of a Most Efficacious Medicine for Soreness, Weakness, and Several Other Distempers of the Eyes* (London, 1745).

Small, E., *North American Cornucopia: Top 100 Indigenous Food Plants* (CRC Press, Boca Raton, FL, 2013).

Smith, M., 'William Turner (C. 1508–1568): Physician, Botanist and Theologian', *Journal of Medical Biology* (1999).

Sneddon, A., *Witchcraft and Magic in Ireland* (Palgrave Macmillan. London, 2015).

Spackman, W. F., *An Analysis of the Occupations of the People of the United Kingdom of Great Britain* (William Frederick Spackman, London, 1847).

Spearing, A. C., *Readings in Medieval Poetry* (Cambridge University Press, Cambridge, 1989).

Speeches Delivered to Queen Elizabeth, on Her Visit to Giles Brudges, Lord Chandos , at Sudeley Castle, in Gloucestershire (Johnson & Warwick, London, 1815).

Stobart, A., *Household Medicine in Seventeenth-Century England* (Bloomsbury Academic, London, 2016).

Stopp, H. (ed), *The Cookbook by Sabina Welserin* (University of Heidelberg, Germany, 1980)

Strickland, A., *Lives of the Queens of England* (George Bell & Sons, London, 1884).

Strybel, M & R. Strybel, *Polish Heritage Cookery* (Hippocrene Books, New York, 1993).

Tansley, A. G. 'Arthur Harry Church. 1865-1937', Obituary Notices of Fellows of the Royal Society, Vol. 2, No. 7 (1939).

Pepys, S., *The Diary of Samuel Pepys, Complete 1664* (Good Press, Glasgow, 2019).

The Homeopathic Recorder Vol. IV (Boericke & Tafel, Philadelphia, PA, 1889).

The Old Bailey, Ref: t18261026-215.

The Old Bailey, Ref: t18481023-2442.

Thomas, K., *Religion and the Decline of Magic* (Penguin, London, 2003).

Thompson, C. J., *The Apothecary in England from the Thirteenth to the Close of the Sixteenth Century* (Proceedings of the Royal Society of Medicine, London, 1915).

Thomson, A., *The London Dispensatory* (Longman, Hurst, Rees, Orme & Brown, London, 1815).

Thoreau, H. D., *The Man Himself* (Musaicum Books, ebook, 2017).

Thorndike, L., *A History of Magic and Experimental Science* Vol. 1 (Columbia University Press, New York & London, 1923).

Tildesley, N. T. et al., Salvia Lavandulaefolia (Spanish Sage) Enhances Memory in Healthy Young Volunteers, *Pharmacology Biochemistry and Behaviour* Vol. 75, Issue 3 (June (2003).

Titley, N. M. (trans), *The Ni'matnama Manuscript of the Sultans of Mandu* (Routledge, London, 2004).

Turner, W., *The First and Seconde Partes of the Herbal of William Turner* (Arnold Birckman, 1568).

Tusser, T., *Five Hundred Pointes of Good Husbandrie* (Trubner & Co, London, 1878).

Veenker, R., A, *The Biblical Archaeologist*, Vol 44, no.4, (1981).

Vickery, R, *Vickery's Folk Flora* (Weidenfeld & Nicolson, London, 2019).

Von Bingen, Hildegard & P. Throop (illus), *Hildegard von Bingen's Physica* (Healing Arts Press, Rochester, VT, 1998).

Von Nettesheim, Agrippa H. C., *The Philosophy of Natural Magic* (Jazzybee Verlag Jurgen Beck, 2014).

Von Störck, Anton, *Observations Upon a Treatise on the Virtues of Hemlock* (J. Meres, London, 1761).

W. M., *The Compleat Cook* (Nath Brook, London, 1658).

Walafrid, S., *On the Cultivation of Gardens. A Ninth Century Gardening Book* (Ithuriel"s Spear, San Francisco, CA, 2009).

Walcott Emmart, E., *Concerning the Badianus Manuscript, an Aztec Herbal, 'Codex Barberini, Latin 241'* (The Smithsonian Institute, Washington,1935).

Walton, I., *The Complete Angler* (C. & C. Whittingham, London, 1826).

Weiss Adamson, M. (ed.), *Food in the Middle Ages* (Taylor & Francis, Oxford, 1995).

Wexler, P. (ed.), *Toxicology in Antiquity* (Elsevier, London & New York, 2019).

Whaley, L., *Women and the Practice of Medical Care in Early Modern Europe, 1400–1800* (Palgrave Macmillan, London, 2011).

Wheeler, K., *A Natural History of Nettles* (Trafford, Canada, 2007).

Wilde, O., I. Small (ed.). *The Complete Works of Oscar Wilde* (Oxford University Press, Oxford & New York, 2005).

Williamson, G. C., *Lady Anne Clifford, Countess of Dorset, Pembroke & Montgomery, 1590–1676* (Titus Wilson & Son, Kendal, 1922).

Woodville, W., *Medical Botany Containing Systematic and General Descriptions with Plates* (James Phillips, London, 1790).

Woolf, J, *Women's Business: 17th Century Female Pharmacists* (Science History Institute, Philadelphia, PA, 2009).

Woolley, B., *The Herbalist. Nicholas Culpeper and the Fight for Medical Freedom* (Harper Collins, London, 2012).

World Health Organization, *Global Report on Traditional and Complementary Medicine* (WHO, Luxembourg, 2019).

World Health Organization, *Legal Status of Traditional Medicine and Complementary/ Alternative Medicine: Worldwide Review* (WHO, Geneva, 2001).

Wright, P. (ed.), *The Poems of John Keats* (Wordsworth Editions Ltd, Hertfordshire, 1994).

Websites

BBC News, 30 March 2015, *1,000-year-old onion and garlic eye remedy kills MRSA*, www.bbc.co.uk/news/uk-england-nottinghamshire-32117815 (accessed 10 June 2021).

BBC News, 2011, Babbs, H, *London's history of herbal treatments*, www.bbc.co.uk/news/ uk-england-london-13713424 (accessed 20 June 2021).

Cook, E. (trans), *Maistre Chiquart, Du fait de cuisine*, www.daviddfriedman.com/ Medieval/Cookbooks/Du_Fait_de_Cuisine/Du_fait_de_Cuisine.html, (accessed 14 June 2021).

Cox, N. & K. Dannehl, 'Hearing horn – Hellebore', *Dictionary of Traded Goods and Commodities 1550–1820* (Wolverhampton, 2007), *British History Online* www. british-history.ac.uk/no-series/traded-goods-dictionary/1550-1820/hearing-horn-hellebore (accessed 21 June 2021).

Cox, N. & K. Dannehl, 'Hemp – Herse', *Dictionary of Traded Goods and Commodities 1550–1820* (Wolverhampton, 2007), *British History Online*, www.british-history. ac.uk/no-series/traded-goods-dictionary/1550-1820/hemp-herse (accessed 28 June 2021).

Cox, N. & K. Dannehl, 'Caracca nut – Carduus water', *Dictionary of Traded Goods and Commodities 1550–1820* (Wolverhampton, 2007), *British History Online*, www. british-history.ac.uk/no-series/traded-goods-dictionary/1550-1820/caracca-nut-carduus-water (accessed 12 February 2021).

Cox, N. & K. Dannehl, 'Valencia almond – Vermilion', *Dictionary of Traded Goods and Commodities 1550-1820* (Wolverhampton, 2007), *British History Online*, www.british-history.ac.uk/no-series/traded-goods-dictionary/1550-1820/valencia-almond-vermilion (accessed 13 February 2021).

De Monmarché, G. (trans), *Le Recueil de Riom*, www.erminespot.com/wp-content/uploads/2009/01/le-recueil-de-riom.pdf (accessed on 13 May 2021).

Du Libre B, from *Due Libri di Cucina*, www.daviddfriedman.com/Medieval/Cookbooks/Due_Libre_B/Due_Libre_B.pdf (accessed, 15, June 2021).

Duncan Napier's Diary Records, https://amp.ww.en.freejournal.org/13497030/1/duncan-napier.html (accessed 20 April 2021).

Forest, M. (trans), *Koge Bog* (Cook book), (Salomone Sartorio, Copenhagen, 1616), www.forest.gen.nz/Medieval/articles/cooking/1616.html (accessed, 20 May 2021).

Friedman, D. (trans), *The Cookbook of Sabrina Welserin*, www.daviddfriedman.com/Medieval/Cookbooks/Sabrina_Welserin.html, (accessed 20 May 2021).

Gomes, F. (trans), *A Treatise of Portuguese Cuisine from the 15th Century* (2007), www.medievalcookery.com/notes/tratado.html (accessed 1 May 2021).

Herbal medicine market size and forecast, by product (tablets & capsules, powders, extracts), by indication (digestive disorders, respiratory disorders, blood disorders), and trend analysis, 2014–2024 (2017, Market Research Report, Hexa Research), www.hexaresearch.com/research-report/global-herbal-medicine-market (accessed on 2 March 2021).

Kitab al-Tabeekh fi 'l-Maghrib wa 'l-Andalus fi 'Asr al-Muwahhidin (The Cookbook of al-Maghrib and Andalusia in the era of the Almohads), http://daviddfriedman.com/Medieval/Cookbooks/Andalusian/andalusian7.htm#Heading360 (accessed 13 May 2021).

Kovacs, B. (trans), *The Prince of Transylvania's Court Master Chef.* Glenn Gorsuch (ed.), *The Prince of Transylvania's Court Cookbook, from the 16th Century. The Science of Cooking*, www.medievalcookery.com/etexts/transylvania-v2.pdf (accessed 27 April 2021).

Lee, M. R, *The Solanaceae II: The Mandrake; in League with the Devil* (J. R. College of Physicians, Edinburgh, 2006, Vol. 36), www.rcpe.ac.uk/journal/issue/journal_36_3/W_Lee_2.pdf (accessed 3 May 2021)

Leong, E., *Making Medicines in the Early Modern Household*, Bulletin of the History of Medicine, Vol. 82, No.1 (2008) www.jstor.org/stable/44448509?read-now=1&refreqid=excelsior%3Afb4a0bd167d8336ff464b10fe1473f04&seq=19#page_scan_tab_contents (accessed 14 April 2021).

Libre del Coch, 1529, www.florilegium.org/files/FOOD-MANUSCRIPTS/Guisados1-art.html (accessed, 24 April 2021).

Mahomoodally, M., *Traditional Medicines in Africa: An Appraisal of Ten Potent African Medicinal Plants* (Hindawi, 2013), www.who.int/mediacentre/news/releases/release38/en/ (accessed 30 May 2021).

Muusers, C. (trans), *Wel ende edelike spijse* (Good and noble food), www.coquinaria.nl/kooktekst/Edelikespijse0.htm (accessed on 6 May 2021).

Oxford Botanic Garden, www.obga.ox.ac.uk/1648-collection (accessed 5 April 2021).

Pegge, S. (ed.), *Forme of Cury: A Roll of Ancient English Cookery. Compiled, about A.D. 1390, by the Master-Cooks of King RICHARD II* (1780), www.gutenberg.org/cache/epub/8102/pg8102.html (accessed 24 February 2021).

Pelling, M. & F. White, 'JACKSON, Elizabeth', in *Physicians and Irregular Medical Practitioners in London 1550–1640 Database* (London, 2004), *British History Online*, www.british-history.ac.uk/no-series/london-physicians/1550-1640/jackson-elizabeth (accessed 26 March 2021).

Pelling, M. & F. White, 'ACTOUR, John', in *Physicians and Irregular Medical Practitioners in London 1550–1640 Database* (London, 2004), *British History Online*, www.british-history.ac.uk/no-series/london-physicians/1550-1640/actour-john (accessed 26 March 2021).

Pelling, M. & F. White, 'ANTHONY, Francis', in *Physicians and Irregular Medical Practitioners in London 1550–1640 Database* (London, 2004), *British History Online*, www.british-history.ac.uk/no-series/london-physicians/1550-1640/anthony-francis (accessed 26 March 2021).

Pelling, M. & F. White, 'AUDLING, Edward', in *Physicians and Irregular Medical Practitioners in London 1550–1640 Database* (London, 2004), *British History Online*, www.british-history.ac.uk/no-series/london-physicians/1550-1640/audling-edward (accessed 26 March 2021).

Pelling, M. & F. White, 'DESILAR, Matthew', in *Physicians and Irregular Medical Practitioners in London 1550–1640 Database* (London, 2004), *British History Online*, www.british-history.ac.uk/no-series/london-physicians/1550-1640/desilar-matthew (accessed 26 March 2021).

Pelling, M. & F. White, 'GLORIANA, Susanna', in *Physicians and Irregular Medical Practitioners in London 1550–1640 Database* (London, 2004), *British History Online* www.british-history.ac.uk/no-series/london-physicians/1550-1640/gloriana-susanna (accessed 26 March 2021).

Perry, C. (trans), *An Anonymous Andalusian Cookbook of the 13th Century*, http://daviddfriedman.com/Medieval/Cookbooks/Andalusian/andalusian_contents.htm (accessed 15 June 2021).

Prescott, J. (trans), *Le Viandier de Taillevent* (Alfarhaugr Publishing Society, Oregon, 1989), www.telusplanet.net/public/prescotj/data/viandier/viandier4.html (accessed 20 February 2021).

Rooibos and Buchu lamb shanks, https://static1.squarespace.com/static/564312 e0e4b02d0ff72509f3/t/5e7da228b4d27021652c94df/1585292816689/ Rooibos+lamb+shank (accessed, 20 April 2021).

Sengoku Daimyo, 2019 https://sengokudaimyo.com/rm-ch12 (accessed, 22 May,2021)

Senn, C. H., *The Book of Sauces* (Applewood Books, Massachusetts, 1915).

Spitalfields Life, *The Nine Herb Charm*, https://spitalfieldslife.com/2018/05/15/the-nine-herbs-charm/ (accessed 2 February 2021).

Summers, Montague (trans), *The Malleus Maleficarum* (1928) www.sacred-texts.com/pag/mm/index.htm (accessed 22 March 2021).

The Japanese Pharmacopoeia, 17th Edition (2016), www.mhlw.go.jp/file/06-Seisakujouhou-11120000-Iyakushokuhinkyoku/JP17_REV_1.pdf (accessed 3 June 2021).